Occupational English Test: Preparation Book

Reading Sub-test

Volume 2

By Anna Hartford

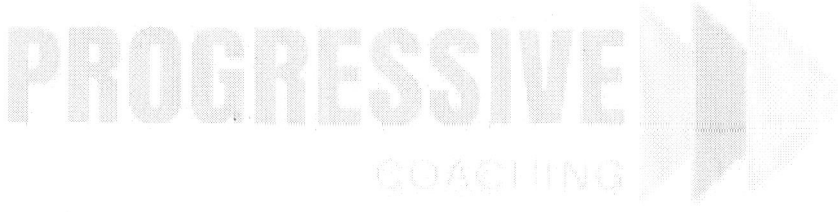

Table of Contents

Introduction

Welcome to Volume 2 of the Reading Sub-test series.

This book was written for candidates across the world taking the Occupational English Test (OET), to provide guidance, tips and practice that will make the OET easier to pass and less stressful.

The content of this book is based on the author's many years of experience in preparing candidates for the OET. It includes advice for preparation that has been tried and tested by candidates from a wide variety of backgrounds and levels of English ability.

The first volume in this series (Reading Sub-test: Volume 1) introduced you to the basic approaches to preparing for the Reading Sub-test, as well as some helpful test-taking strategies. This volume (Volume 2) will continue to prepare you, by increasing your proficiency in the English language and confidence with the medical vocabulary used in the Reading Sub-test.

There are 3 main areas covered in Volume 2 of this series. These are:

1. Knowing how to guess the meaning of unknown words

2. Familiarity with common medical terms

3. Practice tests

The first part, guessing unknown words, will show you how to use the context and structure of words you don't know the meaning of to guess their meaning to the best of your ability.

The second part, common medical terms, provides you with a comprehensive list of the most useful medical terminology to revise before the test. Revising this list will give you a solid foundation of medical English vocabulary.

The third part of this volume consists of 3 new practice tests, different to the practice tests from volume 1. This will allow you to continue practicing test-taking strategies and vocabulary skills in a setting that simulates the OET. The practice tests also feature answer keys and guides to help you understand why each answer is correct and where it comes from.

I wish you the best of luck with your preparation!

- Anna Hartford
(10 Sept 2018)

Part 1: Guessing Unknown Words

Using Context

When you guess the meaning of a word by using its context, you need to consider first the *immediate* context. The immediate context means the other words in the same sentence.

If this is not enough for you to guess the word's meaning, then you need to use the *wider* context. The wider context is the sentences which come before and after the one which contains the word you are guessing.

Immediate context

Consider the following example:

> "Although your blood pressure has responded well to the medication, your high-sugar, high-fat diet and lack of physical activity will continue to put the health of your cardiovascular system in a disadvantageous position."

Imagine that the word you are trying to guess is 'disadvantageous'. The *immediate* context of the word gives you the following information:
- It is probably an adjective, because it comes before a noun ('position')
- It is probably negative, because:
  - It relates to 'high-fat diet, which is a bad thing, AND
  - Because the sentence begins with 'although', a contrast marker (so, the idea in the second clause contrasts with the first clause, which is positive: 'responded well' is good for the blood pressure).

A good guess for the meaning of this word at this point would be 'bad'. This is probably close enough for you to understand the main idea, and be able to keep reading.

Wider context

Now consider the following paragraph:

> "Although your blood pressure has responded well to the medication, your high-sugar, high-fat diet and lack of physical activity will continue to put the health of your cardiovascular system in a disadvantageous position. This is why you had an infarction of the heart muscle, which caused the heart to stop working properly."

Imagine the word you want to guess this time is '**infarction**'. The *immediate* context of the word does not tell you much. It is clearly a noun (because it has "an" in front of it), but it is difficult to determine more than this using only the sentence that the word occurs in.

To guess the meaning, you need to use the *wider* context, i.e. the sentences which come before and after. Using the wider context, you can tell the following:

- It is probably negative, because it is the result of the cardiovascular system being in a 'disadvantageous (bad) position'.
- It led to the heart not working properly.

From this, you can guess that the word means something like 'disease' or 'death' (because the heart doesn't work anymore).

Using prefixes, suffixes and roots

First, it's important to know what prefixes, roots and suffixes are. The definitions of these terms are provided:

- **Prefix:** a term placed at the beginning of a word, to modify or change its meaning ("pre" means "before").
- **Root:** the middle part of a word.
- **Suffix:** the ending part of a word, that modifies the meaning of the word.

Now, consider the following sentence:

> "Although your blood pressure has responded well to the medication, your high-sugar, high-fat diet and lack of physical activity will continue to put the health of your cardiovascular system in a disadvantageous position."

Imagine (again) that the word you want to guess in this sentence is **'disadvantageous'**. This word can be broken down into three components:

- *dis-* (the prefix)
- *advantage* (the root) and
- *-ous* (the suffix).

You can get the following information by studying the word in this way:

- It is probably an adjective, because it ends in *-ous*, which is a common suffix for adjectives
- It is probably negative, because it begins with a negative prefix *dis-*
- Its meaning is probably opposite to the root of the word, *advantage*

As before, a good guess for the word at this point would be 'bad'. Again, this would be close enough to allow you to understand the main idea of the text and keep reading.

Here is an example of how we can use a prefix, root and suffix to guess the meaning of an unfamiliar, but more *medical* word.

Let's pretend that the word you are trying to guess the meaning of is "**achondroplasia**".

This word is composed of the following terms:
- Prefix: a- (definition: no, not, without)
- Root: -chondro- (definition: cartilage)
- Suffix: -plasia (definition: development, formation)

If you know the definition of the prefix, root and suffix, you can therefore guess (correctly) that the meaning of "achondroplasia" is "no cartilage development" or "no cartilage formation".

Part 2: Useful Medical Terms

In the Reading Sub-test, it can be very helpful to know the meaning of common terms that are used as prefixes, roots and suffixes in medical terminology. This will make it easier for you to guess the meaning of unfamiliar words. The example given in Part 1, "achondroplasia", provides a good demonstration of how helpful it can be to familiarise yourself with common medical prefixes, roots and suffixes.

In the tables to follow, you are provided with a list of common prefixes and suffixes used in a healthcare context.

Please note, that any prefix or suffix can also be used as a root. For example, the prefix "glyc" (meaning glucose or sugar) can be used as a prefix in the word "glycolysis" or a root in the word "hyperglycemia".

Commonly used medical prefixes:

Prefix	Meaning	Example and Definition
a/an-	No, not, without	Anuria (no urination)
abdomin(o)-	Abdomen	Abdominal (relating to the abdomen)
acoust-	Hearing, sound	Acoustic (relating to sound or the sense of hearing)
adip-	Fat	Adipose tissue (fat tissue)
adren-	Adrenal gland	Adrenaline (a hormone secreted by the adrenal glands)
aer-	Air	Aerated (made effervescent by adding air)
angio-	Blood vessel	Angiogenesis (the development of new blood vessels)
anti-	Against	Antiviral (effective against viruses)

arterio-	Artery	Arteriosclerosis (thickening and hardening of the walls of the arteries)
arthr-	Joint	Arthritis (a disease causing painful inflammation and stiffness of the joints)
athero-	Plaque (fatty substance)	Atherosclerosis (a disease of the arteries characterized by the deposition of fatty material on their inner walls)
auto-	Self, own	Autoimmune (relating to disease caused by antibodies or lymphocytes produced against substances naturally present in the body)
bar(o)-	Weight	Bariatric (relating to weight or obesity)
bi-	Two	Biphasic (having two phases)
brachi(o)-	Arm	Brachial artery (the major blood vessel of the upper arm)
brachy-	Short	Brachydactyly (short fingers or toes)
brady-	Slow	Bradycardia (abnormally slow heart action)
bronch(o)-	Bronchial tube	Bronchoscopy (an endoscopic technique of visualizing the inside of the airways)
burs-	Bursa (a sack of fluid near a joint)	Bursitis (inflammation of the bursae)
carcin(o)-	Cancer, cancerous	Carcinoma (a cancer arising in the epithelial tissue)

cardi(o)-	Heart	Carditis (inflammation of the heart tissue)
cephal-	Head	Cephalic (relating to the head)
cerebr(o)-	Cerebrum (largest part of brain)	Cerebral (relating to the cerebrum)
cerebell(o)-	Cerebellum	Cerebellar (relating to the cerebellum)
cervic(o)-	Neck	Cervical (relating to the neck)
chem(o)-	Chemical, drug-related	Chemotherapy (the treatment of disease using chemical substances)
chol-	Bile, Gall	Cholangitis (an infection of the bile duct)
chondr(o)-	Cartilage	Chondroblast (cells which form chondrocytes in the cartilage matrix)
circum-	Around	Circumduction (movement of a limb or extremity so that the distal end describes a circle)
colp(o)-	Vagina	Colposcopy (a procedure to closely examine the cervix and vagina)
comat(o)-	Deep sleep, coma	Comatose (relating to or in a state of coma)
contus(o)-	Bruise	Contusion (a bruise)
contra-	Against, opposite	Contraindication (a condition or circumstance which suggests that a technique/drug should not be used)

cost(o)-	Rib	Costal cartilage (a segment of cartilage that connects the sternum to the ribs)
cortico-	Cortex, outer region	Corticobulbar tract (a motor pathway connecting the motor cortex to the Medullary pyramids)
crani(o)-	Skull	Craniotomy (surgical removal of a portion of the skull)
cry(o)-	Cold, freezing	Cryoablation (the medical use of extreme cold to destroy tissue)
cutane(o)-	Skin	Cutaneous (related to the skin)
cyt(o)-	Cell	Cytology (the study of plant or animal cells)
de-	Lack of, down, less, removal of	Debridement (the removal of damaged tissue or foreign objects from a wound)
dec-	Ten	Decade (a period of 10 years)
dent(o)-	Tooth, teeth	Dentition (the arrangement or condition of the teeth)
derm(o)-	Skin	Dermatology (the branch of medicine concerned with skin disorders)
dextr(o)-	Right	Dextrocardia (a rare congenital condition in which the apex of the heart is located on the right-hand side of the body)
dipl(o)-	Double	Diplopia (double vision)
dips(o)-	Thirst	Hyperdipsia (excessive thirst)

dors(o)-	Back (of the body)	Dorsal (related to the back of the body)
dys-	Bad, painful, difficult, abnormal	Dyspepsia (painful digestion)
ectro-	Congenital absence	Ectrodactylism (congenital absence of all or part of one or more fingers or toes)
encephal(o)-	Brain	Encephalitis (inflammation of the brain)
enter(o)-	Intestines	Enteropathy (a disease of the intestine)
epi-	Above, upon, on	Epidermis (the surface epithelium of the skin)
equi-	Equality, equal	Equidistant (at equal distances)
erythem(o)-	Red, flushed	Erythematous (red, due to dilatation and congestion of the capillaries)
eu-	Good, normal	Euthyroid (having a normally functioning thyroid gland)
ex-/extra-	Outside, away from	Extracorporeal (outside of the body)
fibr(o)-	Fibre	Fibromuscular (relating to fibre and muscular tissue)
ferr(o)-	Iron	Ferritin (a protein that stores iron in the tIssue)
fet(o)-	Fetus	Fetal (relating to a fetus)
follicul(o)-	Follicle, small sac	Folliculitis (inflammation of the hair follicles)

fore-	In front, foremost	Foregut (the anterior part of the gut, towards the mouth)
galact(o)-	Milk	Galactorrhea (a milky nipple discharge)
gastr(o)-	Stomach	Gastric reflux (a long-term condition where stomach contents come back up into the esophagus)
gingiv(o)-	Gum	Gingivitis (inflammation of the gums)
gluc(o)- OR glyc(o)-	Glucose, sugar	Hyperglycemia (high blood sugar level)
gonad(o)-	Sex glands	Gonadotropin (a hormone which stimulates the activity of the sex glands)
gynaec(o)-	Female, woman	Gynaecology (the branch of medicine which deals with functions and diseases specific to females)
hem(o)- OR hemat(o)-	Blood	Hemolysis (the rupture or destruction of red blood cells)
hepat(o)-	Liver	Hepatic flexure (the bend in the colon on the right side of the body near the liver)
hemi-	Half	Hemiplegia (paralysis of one side of the body)
hidr(o)-	Sweat	Hyperhidrosis (excessive sweating)
hist(o)-	Tissue	Histological (relating to tissues seen under a microscope)

home(o)-	Same, constant, unchanging	Homeostasis (a stable, physiological state of equilibrium)
hydr(o)-	Water	Hydration (the process of ingesting/absorbing water)
hyper-	Above, excessive	Hypertension (high blood pressure)
hyp(o)-	Deficient, low, less than normal	Hypothermia (low body temperature)
infra-	Below, beneath	Infraorbital (beneath the orbit)
inter-	Between	Intergenerational (present between more than one generation)
intra-	Within	Intrauterine (within the uterus)
ipsi-	Same	Ipsilateral (on the same side)
juxta-	Near	Juxtaglomerular (next to the glomerulus in the kidney)
jaund-	Yellow	Jaundice (a yellow discolouration of the skin)
kal-	Potassium	Hypokalemia (low serum potassium)
kinesi(o)-	Movement	Kinesiology (the study of the mechanics of body movements)
kyph-	Humpback	Kyphosis (excessive outward curvature of the spine, causing hunching of the back)
lacrim(o)-	Tear, tear duct, lacrimal duct	Lacrimation (the flow of tears)

lact(o)-	Milk	Lactation (the secretion of milk by the mammary glands)
lapar(o)-	Abdomen	Laparoscopy (a surgical procedure in which a fibre-optic instrument is inserted through the abdominal wall)
lept(o)-	Thin, slender	Leptomeninges (the inner two meninges, the arachnoid and the pia mater)
leuk(o)-	White	Leukocyte (white blood cell)
ligat(o)-	Binding, tying	Ligation (the surgical procedure of tying a ligature around a blood vessel, duct or tube in the body)
lingu(o)-	Tongue	Lingula (a tongue-shaped process or part)
lip(o)-	Fat, lipid	Liposuction (removal of excess fat from under the skin by suction)
lith(o)-	Stone, calculus	Cholelith (solid material that forms in the gallbladder or common bile duct, gallstone)
macro-	Large	Fetal macrosomia (diagnosis for a newborn who's significantly larger than average)
mal-	Bad	Malodorous (smelling very unpleasant)
mamm(o)- OR mast(o)-	Breast	Mammography (a technique using X-rays to diagnose and locate tumours of the breasts)
medi(o)-	Middle	Mediastinum (the middle part of the chest)

mega-	Large	Megacardia (an abnormal enlargement of the heart)
meta-	Change, beyond	Metamorphosis (a change of the form or nature of a thing or person into a different one)
mono-	One	Monoamine (a compound having a single amine group in its molecule, e.g. serotonin, noradrenaline)
nat-	Birth	Prenatal (before birth)
natr-	Sodium	Hyponatremia (low serum sodium level)
necro-	Death	Necrosis (death of body tissues)
neo-	New	Neonate (newborn baby)
nephr(o)-	Kidney	Nephrotoxic (poisonous to the kidneys)
neur(o)-	Nerve	Neurotransmitter (a chemical substance which is released at the end of a nerve fibre)
noci-	Relating to harm, injury or pain	Nociceptor (a sensory receptor for painful stimuli)
nulli-	None	Nulliparity (the condition of never having given birth)
obstetr(o)-	Pregnancy	Obstetrics (the branch of medicine and surgery concerned with childbirth and midwifery)

ocul(o)-	Eye	Oculomotor (relating to the motion of the eye)
odyn(o)-	Pain	Odynophagia (pain on swallowing food and fluids)
olig(o)-	Sparse, few	Oliguria (the production of abnormally small amounts of urine)
onc(o)-	Cancer, tumour	Oncology (the study and treatment of tumours)
onych(o)-	Nail (of fingers or toes)	Onychomycosis (a fungal infection of the nail)
ophthalm(o)-	Eye, vision	Ophthalmology (the branch of medicine concerned with the study and treatment of disorders and diseases of the eye)
oste(o)-	Bone	Osteoporosis (a medical condition in which the bones become brittle and fragile from loss of tissue)
ot(o)-	Ear	Otoscope (an instrument designed for visual examination of the eardrum and outer ear)
pan-	All	Pancytopenia (deficiency of all three cellular components of the blood: red cells, white cells, and platelets)
para-	Near, beside, abnormal	Paraplegia (paralysis of both of the legs and lower body)

path-	Disease	Pathology (the science of the causes and effects of diseases)
ped(o)-	Child, foot	Tinea pedis (a fungal infection of the feet)
peri-	Surrounding	Pericarditis (inflammation of the membrane surrounding the heart)
pharmac(o)-	Drug	Pharmacology (the uses, effects, and modes of action of drugs)
pharmaceut(o)-	Drug	Pharmaceutical (relating to medicinal drugs, or their preparation, use, or sale)
phlebo-	Vein	Phlebotomy (the surgical opening or puncture of a vein)
phot(o)-	Light	Photosensitivity (sensitivity to light)
ple(o)-	Many, more	Pleomorphism (the occurrence of many different forms of an object, such as cells in a tumour)
pneum-	Lung, air, gas	Pneumothorax (the presence of air or gas in the cavity between the lungs and the chest wall)
poly-	Many, much	Polycythemia (an abnormally increased concentration of haemoglobin in the blood)
post-	After, behind	Postmortem (an examination of a dead body to determine the cause of death)
poster(o)-	Back (of the body), behind	Posterior (further back in position, of or nearer the rear)

pre-	Before, in front of	Premature (of a baby: born before the end of the full term of gestation)
primi-	First	Primigravida (a woman who is pregnant for the first time)
pro-	Before, forward	Progenitor (an ancestor or parent)
pseudo-	False	Pseudocapsule (a structure, similar to a capsule, that surrounds some carcinomas)
pulmon-	Lung	Pulmonary (relating to the lungs)
purul(o)-	Pus	Purulent (consisting of, containing, or discharging pus)
py(o)-	Pus	Pyogenic (involving or relating to the production of pus)
pyrex(o)-	Fever	Pyrexia (raised body temperature, fever)
quadri-	Four, square	Quadrivalent (having a valency of four)
quart-	Fourth, four	Quarter (one fourth)
radi(o)-	X-rays, radioactivity, radius (a lower arm bone)	Radiolucent (transparent to X-rays)
respir(o)-	Breath	Respiration (the action of breathing)
resuscit(o)-	To revive	Resuscitation (the action or process of reviving someone)
retro-	Behind, back, backward	Retropulsion (an abnormal tendency to walk backwards)

rhin(o)-	Nose	Rhinitis (inflammation of the mucous membrane of the nose)
semi-	Half	Semipermeable (allowing certain substances to pass through it but not others)
seps(o)-	Infection	Sepsis (the presence in tissues of harmful bacteria and their toxins)
sept(o)-	Partition	Septum (a partition separating two chambers)
spir(o)-	To breathe	Spirometry (a test of pulmonary function by measuring the movement of air in and out of the lungs)
sten(o)-	Narrowed, constricted	Stenosis (the abnormal narrowing of a passage in the body)
sub-	Under, below	Suboptimal (less than optimal)
super-	Above, beyond	Superimposed (placed over or on top of another)
supra-	Above, upper	Suprascapular (on the upper part of the scapula)
sym- OR syn-	Together, with	Symbiosis (Interaction between two different organisms living in close physical association)
tachy-	Fast	Tachycardia (an abnormally rapid heart rate)

therm(o)-	Heat	Thermogenic (tending to produce heat)
thorac(o)-	Chest	Thoracic vertebra (each of the twelve bones of the spinal column to which the ribs are attached)
thromb(o)-	Clot	Thrombus (a blood clot formed in the vascular system of the body)
tox(o)- OR toxic(o)-	Poison	Toxicology (the branch of medicine concerned with poisons)
trans-	Across, through	Transition (the process of changing from one state or condition to another)
tri-	Three	Triangle (a plane figure with three straight sides and three angles)
ultra-	Beyond, excess	Ultrasound (a sound having very high frequency)
uni-	One	Unilateral (relating to one side)
ur(o)-	Urine, urinary tract	Urology (the study of the function and disorders of the urinary system)
ureter(o)-	Ureter	Ureteric (relating to the ureters)
urethr(o)-	Urethra	Urethritis (inflammation of the urethra)
uter(o)-	Uterus (womb)	Uterine (relating to the uterus)
valv(o)- OR valvul(o)-	Valve	Valvulopathy (disease or pathology of the valves)

vascul(o)-	Vessel (blood)	Vasculitis (inflammation of the blood vessels or vasculature)
ven(o)-	Vein	Venous (relating to veins)
ventil(o)-	To aerate, oxygenate	Ventilation (the movement of air into a space)
verruc(i)-	Wart	Verrucous (covered with warts or wart-like projections)
vir(o)-	Virus	Virology (the study of viruses)
viscer(o)-	Internal organs	Visceral (relating to the internal organs)
vit(o)-	Life	Vital (lively, full of energy, essential to life)
xanth(o)-	Yellow	Xanthelasma (yellowish deposits of fat underneath the skin)
xen(o)-	Stranger, foreigner, foreign	Xenophobia (fear of strangers)
zo(o)-	Animals, animal life	Zoonosis (a disease which can be transmitted to humans from animals)

Commonly used medical suffixes:

Term	Meaning	Example and Definition
-agra	Excessive pain	Arthragra (acute, severe joint pain such as that caused by gout)
-algesia	Sensitivity to pain	Hyperalgesia (abnormally heightened sensitivity to pain)
-algia	Pain	Myalgia (pain in a muscle or group of muscles)
-ar(y)	Pertaining to	Pulmonary (relating to the lungs)
-atresia	Occlusion	Gynatresia (occlusion of some part of the female genital tract)
-ase	Enzyme	Amylase (an enzyme that converts starch and glycogen into simple sugars)
-assay	Examination, analysis	Immunoassay (a procedure for detecting or measuring specific antigens or antibodies)
-asthenia	Lack of strength	Myasthenia (a condition causing abnormal weakness of certain muscles)
-blast	Embryonic/immature cell	Erythroblast (an immature erythrocyte)
-blastoma	Immature tumour (cells)	Medulloblastoma (a malignant primary brain tumour)
-capnia	Carbon dioxide	Hypercapnia (elevated carbon dioxide in the blood)
-cele	Hernia	Varicocele (a mass of varicose veins in the spermatic cord)
-centesis	Surgical procedure to remove fluid	Amniocentesis (a process in which amniotic fluid is sampled using a hollow needle inserted into the uterus)
-cidal	Killing	Bactericidal (able to kill bacteria)
-crit	To separate	Hematocrit (an instrument for measuring the ratio of the volume of red blood cells to

		the total volume of blood, typically by centrifugation)
-derma	Skin	Scleroderma (hardening of the skin)
-desis	To bind, tie together	Arthrodesis (surgical immobilization of a joint by fusion of the bones)
-ectasia/-ectasis	Dilation, dilatation, widening	Bronchiectasis (abnormal widening of the bronchi or their branches)
-ectomy	Removal, excision, resection	Tonsillectomy (surgical removal of the tonsils)
-edema	Swelling	Angioedema (rapid edema, or swelling, of the area beneath the skin or mucosa)
-emesis	Vomiting	Hyperemesis (severe or prolonged vomiting)
-emia	Blood condition	Anemia (a condition in which there is a deficiency of red cells or of haemoglobin)
-emic	Pertaining to a blood condition	Anemic (having a deficiency of red cells or of haemoglobin)
-esis	Action, condition, state of	Emesis (the action of vomiting)
-esthesia	Nervous sensation	Anaesthesia (insensitivity to pain)
-ferent	To carry	Afferent (carrying or carried towards something)
-fication	The process of making	Calcification (the accumulation of calcium salts in a body tissue, such as in the formation of bone)
-form	Resembling the shape of	Fusiform (tapering at both ends, spindle-shaped)
-gen	Substance that produces/forms something	Teratogen (substance that causes malformation of an embryo)
-genesis	Production, formation	Osteogenesis (formation of bone)

-gram	Record, measurement	Electrocardiogram (a record of a person's heartbeat produced by electrocardiography)
-graph	Instrument for recording, measurement	Electrocardiograph (a machine used for electrocardiography)
-gravid	Pregnant	Primigravid (pregnant for the first time)
-ia	Condition	Polycythemia (an abnormally increased concentration of haemoglobin in the blood)
-itis	Inflammation	Prostatitis (inflammation of the prostate)
-kinesis	Movement	Dyskinesis (a condition of abnormal muscle movements)
-lapse	To slide, fall, sag	Prolapse (a slipping forward or down of a part or organ of the body)
-lexia	Word, phrase	Dyslexia (a difficulty in learning to read or interpret words, letters, and other symbols)
-listhesis	Slippage	Spondylolisthesis (the slippage of one vertebral body over another)
-logy	The study of something	Cardiology (the branch of medicine that deals with diseases and abnormalities of the heart)
-lucent	Shining, glowing, marked by clarity or translucence	Radiolucent (transparent to X-rays)
-lysis	Breakdown, separation, destruction, loosening	Hemolysis (destruction of red blood cells)
-lytic	To reduce, destroy, separate, breakdown	Osteolytic (pertaining to the dissolution of bone)
-malacia	Softening	Osteomalacia (softening of the bones)
-megaly	Enlargement	Cardiomegaly (abnormal enlargement of the heart)

-oid	Resembling, derived from	Dermoid (resembling skin)
-oma	Tumour	Sarcoma (a malignant tumour of connective tissue)
-opaque	Obscure	Radiopaque (opaque to X-rays or similar radiation)
-opsy	Investigation of, view of	Biopsy (an examination of tissue removed from a living body)
-oxia	Oxygen	Hypoxia (oxygen deficiency)
-parous	Bearing, bringing forth	Multiparous (having borne more than one child)
-paresis	Weakness	Hemiparesis (weakness of one side of the body)
-pareunia	Sexual intercourse	Dyspareunia (painful or uncomfortable sexual intercourse)
-partum	Birth, labour	Postpartum (following childbirth)
-pathy	Disease, emotion	Cardiomyopathy (chronic disease of the heart muscle)
-penia	Deficiency, loss	Sarcopenia (he loss of skeletal muscle mass and strength)
-phage	Eat, swallow	Oligophage (an organism that eats only a few or very specific foods)
-phasia	Speech	Dysphasia (a language disorder marked by deficiency in the generation or comprehension of speech)
-philic	Attracting	Hydrophilic (having a tendency to mix with or dissolve in water)
-phobia	Fear	Agoraphobia (an irrational fear of open or public places)
-phylaxis	Protection	Prophylaxis (treatment given or action taken to prevent disease)

-plasia	Development, formation	Metaplasia (abnormal tissue formation)
-plasm	Structure	Neoplasm (a new growth or structure in the body)
-plastic	Causing development, formation	Neoplastic (causing the formation of a new growth or structure)
-plasty	Surgical repair	Rhinoplasty (surgical repair of the nose)
-plegia OR -plegic	Paralysis, palsy	Quadriplegia (paralysis of all four limbs)
-pnea	Breathing	Orthopnea (shortness of breath that occurs when lying flat)
-poiesis	Formation	Hematopoiesis (the production of blood cells and platelets)
-rrhage	Bursting forth (of blood)	Hemorrhage (an escape of blood from a ruptured blood vessel)
-rrhea	Flow, discharge	Diarrhea (frequent, loose bowel motions)
-schisis	To split	Palatoschisis (a congenital split in the roof of the mouth)
-sclerosis	Hardening	Atherosclerosis (hardening of the arteries due to atheroma formation)
-scope	Instrument for visual examination	Ophthalmoscope (an instrument for inspecting the retina and other parts of the eye)
-scopy	Visual examination	Bronchoscopy (an endoscopic technique of visualizing the inside of the airways)
-stalsis	Contraction	Peristalsis (the constriction and relaxation of the muscles of the intestine)
-stasis	To stop, control, place	Hemostasis (the stopping of a flow of blood)
-stenosis	Tightening, stricture	Arteriostenosis (narrowing of the diameter of an artery)

-stomy	New opening	Laparostomy (surgical opening of the abdominal cavity)
-suppression	To stop	Immunosuppression (the partial or complete suppression of the immune response)
-tension	Pressure	Hypertension (high blood pressure)
-therapy	Treatment	Physiotherapy (the treatment of disease, injury, or deformity by physical methods)
-tropia	To turn	Esotropia (a form of strabismus in which one or both eyes turn inward)
-tic	Pertaining to	Sclerotic (pertaining to sclerosis)
-tomy	Process of cutting	Craniotomy (surgical cutting of the skull)
-trophy	Nourishment, development, growth	Hypertrophy (excessive growth)
-tropin	Something which stimulates, acts on	Corticotropin (a hormone that stimulates the adrenal cortex)
-ule	Little, small	Macule (a small area of skin discoloration)
-uresis	Urination	Enuresis (involuntary urination)
-uria	Urination, a condition of urine	Dysuria (painful or uncomfortable urination)
-version	To turn	Cardioversion (a medical procedure by which an abnormally fast heart rate or other cardiac arrhythmia is converted to a normal rhythm using electricity or drugs)
-volemia	Blood volume	Hypovolemia (abnormally low blood volume)
-ward	In the direction of	Upward (towards the upper direction, up)
-zyme	Enzyme	Lysozyme (an enzyme that destroys certain bacteria)

This page has intentionally been left blank

Part 3: Practice Tests

28

Test 1

Part A

TIME: 15 minutes

- Look at the four texts, **A – D**, in the separate **Text Booklet**.

- For each question, **1 – 20**, look through the texts, **A – D**, to find the relevant information.

- Write your answers on the spaces provided in this **Question Paper**.

- Answer all the questions within the 15-minute time limit.

Osteoporosis: Questions

Questions 1-7

For each of the questions, **1 – 7**, decide which text (**A, B, C** or **D**) the information comes from. You may use any letter more than once.

In which text can you find information about

1 The test used to diagnose osteoporosis? _____

2 What factors affect the likelihood of having osteoporosis? _____

3 The treatments available? _____

4 How osteoporosis is defined? _____

5 The management of osteopenia? _____

6 The proportion of people who have poor bone health? _____

7 Lifestyle approaches that contribute to osteoporosis? _____

Questions 8 – 14

Answer each of the questions, **8 – 14**, with a word or short phrase from one of the texts.

Each answer may include words, numbers or both. Your answers should be correctly spelled.

8   What is a normal result on a bone density test?

_____

9   Why should osteoporosis be managed as early as possible?

_____

10   How many people in NSW and ACT might have osteopenia or osteoporosis?

_____

11   What level of alcohol intake increases the risk of osteoporosis?

_____

12   What is lost in bones when they become osteoporotic?

_____

13   What should you seek from your doctor if you have any risk factors?

_____

14   What minerals should be taken by people with a T score of -3?

_____

Questions 15 – 20

Complete each of the sentences, **15 – 20**, with a word or short phrase from one of the texts.
Each answer may include words, numbers or both. Your answers should be correctly spelled.

The majority of people affected by osteoporosis are _____ **(15)**.

A _____ **(16)** determines whether bones are normal, osteopenic or osteoporotic.

A normal bone density result still means you must ensure adequate calcium, _____ **(17)**.

When bones become _____ **(18)** due to osteoporosis, there is an increased risk of fractures.

Unfortunately, several factors can increase the risk of osteoporosis, including personal history, lifestyle, medications and _____ **(19)**.

Of the _____ **(20)** people aged over 50 in NSW and ACT, about 71% have osteoporosis.

Osteoporosis: Texts

Risk factors for osteoporosis in men

If you have any of the following risk factors, see your doctor for a bone health check:

Personal	Medical conditions	Medications	Lifestyle issues
Family history Previous fracture Loss of height (3cm or more)	Low testosterone Coeliac disease Chronic liver or kidney disease Rheumatoid arthritis Diabetes	Treatments for prostate cancer Glucocorticoids Anti-epilepsy drugs Some anti-depressants	Smoking Excessive alcohol Being inactive Obesity Low body weight

Source: Osteoporosis Australia

How is osteoporosis diagnosed?

Osteoporosis is diagnosed with a bone density scan (i.e. bone density test). The result will indicate if bones are in the range of normal, osteopenia or osteoporosis:

T-score	Result	Meaning
1 to -1	Normal	You should ensure you have adequate calcium, enough Vitamin D and you do regular exercise – these are all important factors for maintaining healthy bones.
-1 to -2.5	Osteopenia	Take immediate action to minimize further bone loss. Your doctor will ensure calcium and Vitamin D levels are adequate and discuss any possible risk factors for osteoporosis. Your doctor will monitor your bone density with a follow-up DXA scan after 1-2 years.
-2.5 or lower	Osteoporosis	Your doctor will start treatment with specific osteoporosis medicines and ensure adequate calcium and Vitamin D levels. Follow up tests to monitor bone health.

Source: Osteoporosis Australia

Text C

> **FAQs**
> What is osteoporosis?
> Osteoporosis is a condition in which bones become fragile, leading to a higher risk of fractures (or breaks) than in normal bone. Osteoporosis occurs when bones lose minerals, such as calcium, more quickly than the body can replace them, leading to a loss of bone thickness (bone mass or density). As a result, bones become thinner and less dense so that even a minor bump or fall can result in a fracture.
> Who gets osteoporosis? Can it be treated?
> Over 1 million Australians have osteoporosis. It affects both men and women and is most common is adults over 50. Osteoporosis can be treated and there a range of medications available in Australia. It is most important that osteoporosis is detected as early as possible to ensure bone health is managed to prevent fractures.
> What is a bone density test?
> A bone density test is a simple scan that measures the density of your bones (usually at the hip and spine). The results of this test show if your bones are in the range of normal, low bone density or osteoporosis. You doctor will review any risk factors you may have for osteoporosis before referring you for a bone density scan. Medicare rebates apply for many (but not all) cases.

Source: Osteoporosis Australia

Text D

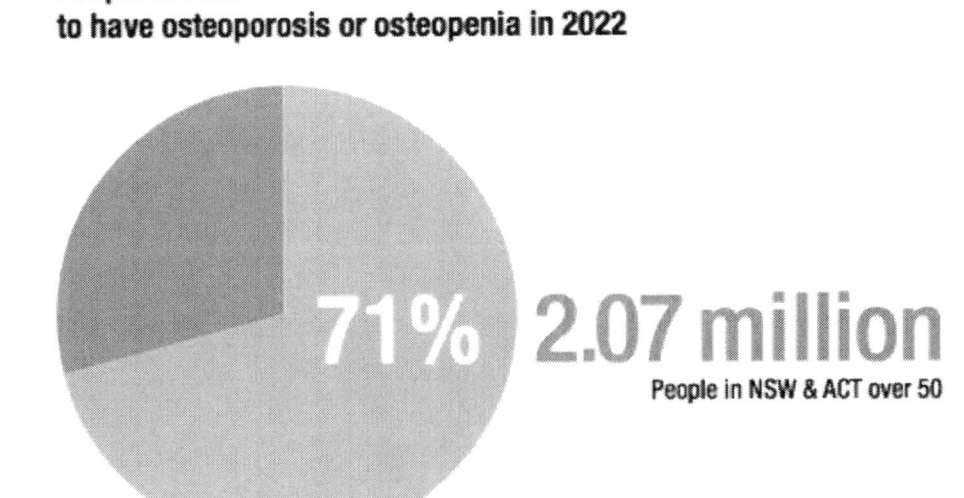

People in NSW & ACT over 50 estimated to have osteoporosis or osteopenia in 2022

71% 2.07 million

People in NSW & ACT over 50

Source: Osteoporosis Australia

END OF PART A
THIS ANSWER BOOKLET WILL BE COLLECTED

Part B

In this part of the test, there are six short extracts relating to the work of health professionals.

For **questions 1 to 6**, choose the answer (**A**, **B** or **C**) which you think fits best according to the text.

---

1. According to the text

   A   Children are vaccinated against three diseases at one year of age

   B   Children under four years cannot receive the diphtheria vaccination

   C   Children receive most of their vaccinations by age 2

Extract from NSW Immunisation Schedule

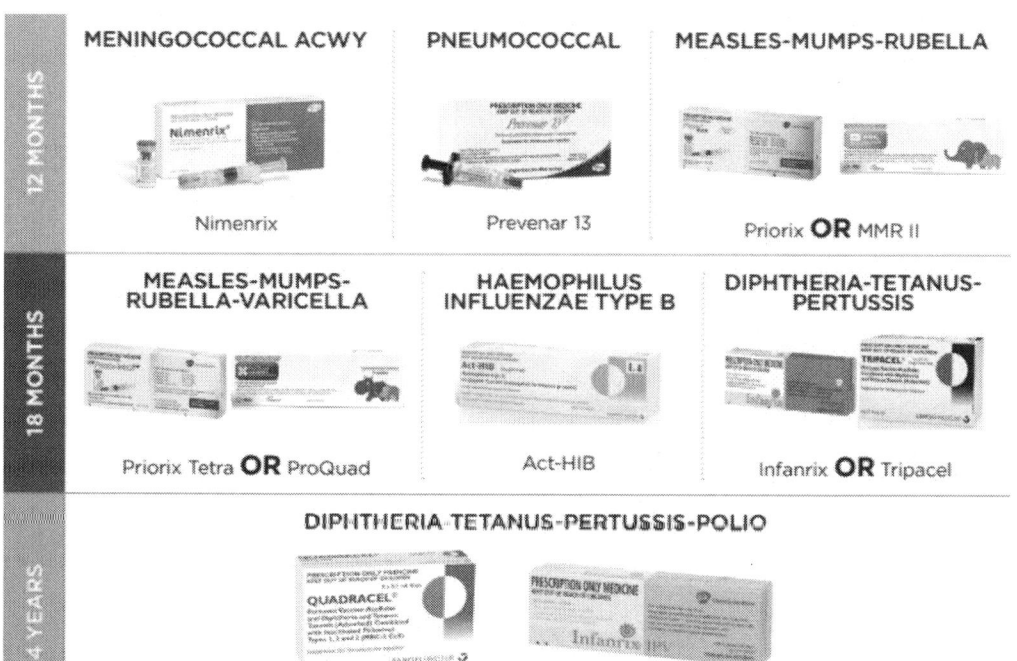

Source: NSW Health (http://www.health.nsw.gov.au/immunisation/Publications/a3-childhood-schedule.pdf)

2. In terms of male hormonal contraception

    A   Men will be able to obtain this through their doctor in the future

    B   Men should become fertile again once they stop it

    C   Men would need two naturally occurring hormones injected

---

Current Research on Hormonal Contraception for Men

A large-scale, international clinical trial of a hormone-based form of male contraception was conducted across seven countries, including Australia, with the support of the World Health Organization (WHO) and CONRAD (connected to Eastern Virginia Medical School, United States).

The study tested a hormone combination treatment to suppress the body's ability to make sperm in a reliable and reversible way. Participants were given an injection of the hormones testosterone and progestogen (a synthetic version of the naturally occurring hormone progesterone) every eight weeks. The study tested how effective this approach was over a 12-month period while carefully monitoring the health of participants. However, this study ended early due to questions about the risks of possible side effects.

Source: Family Planning Victoria (https://www.fpv.org.au/for-you/contraception/long-acting-reversible-contraception-larc/contraceptive-injection-for-men)

3. An addiction can be differentiated from a habit by

    A   The presence or absence of conscious choices

    B   The presence or absence of physical signs

    C   The presence or absence of a person's control over it

---

Addictions and habits

With a habit you are in control of your choices, with an addiction you are not in control of your choices.

- **Addiction** - there is a psychological/physical component; the person is unable to control the aspects of the addiction without help because of the mental or physical conditions involved.

- **Habit** - it is done by choice. The person with the habit can choose to stop, and will subsequently stop successfully if they want to. The psychological/physical dependence is not present.

Addiction, often referred to as *dependency* often leads to *tolerance* - the addicted person needs larger and more regular amounts of whatever they are addicted to in order to receive the same effect. Often, the initial reward is no longer felt, and the addiction continues because withdrawal is so unpleasant.

Source: https://www.medicalnewstoday.com/info/addiction

4. Healthcare staff treating patients taking Clozapine should

    A   Adjust the dosage based on the patient's bowel function

    B   Cease the medication immediately if constipation occurs

    C   Closely monitor the patient's bowel movements

TGA Update: Clozapine and gastrointestinal effects

Clozapine is an atypical antipsychotic agent indicated only in people with treatment-resistant schizophrenia.

The Product Information for clozapine has been updated with information about the potentially fatal risk of intestinal obstruction, faecal impaction and paralytic ileus.

Clozapine-induced gastrointestinal hypomotility (also known as 'slow gut')/impaired intestinal peristalsis can lead to severe constipation and potentially fatal outcomes from faecal impaction, intestinal obstruction, paralytic ileus, megacolon and intestinal ischaemia or infarction.

We recommend close monitoring of bowel function and constipation in patients on clozapine, particularly in patients aged over 60 years and those at higher risk of constipation, such as patients:

- who are taking medications known to cause constipation (anticholinergics)

- with a history of bowel disease

- who have had bowel surgery.

Please note that clozapine is also contraindicated in patients with paralytic ileus.

Source: https://www.tga.gov.au/publication-issue/medicines-safety-update-volume-9-number-2-june-2018#a3

5. Healthcare staff working in operating theatres should

    A   Schedule regular sterilization of reusable medical instruments

    B   Avoid gross contamination of medical instruments when possible

    C   Know that reprocessing contaminated instruments is time consuming

Health care professionals can have a significant impact on the prevention of health care acquired infections or transmission of infection from contaminated instruments. The manner in which medical devices are cared for during and following use can affect the ability for the instruments to be cleaned. Keeping instruments free from gross soiling and minimising the time between instruments leaving the operating rooms and cleaning will reduce the risk of biological material drying on the instrument and becoming lodged in grooves and crevices. Recognition that the reprocessing of complex and difficult to clean medical devices is time consuming and factoring this time into the scheduling of procedures will have a positive effect on the quality outcomes of the cleaning, disinfection and sterilization process, as it will eliminate the need for CSSD and the TSSU and operating room personnel to compromise Standard Operating Procedures in order to deliver the reprocessed devices in time for scheduled procedures.

Source: https://www.tga.gov.au/sites/default/files/report-ncctg-reusable-phr-0405.pdf

6. Regarding the levels of Vitamin D required

    A   The needs of most adults necessitate supplementation during winter

    B   The needs of most adults decrease with increasing age

    C   The needs of most adults can be met through adequate sun exposure

---

Recommended Intake of Vitamin D

Vitamin D intake can be measured in two ways: in micrograms (mcg) and International Units (IU). One microgram of vitamin D is equal to 40 IU of vitamin D. The recommended intakes of vitamin D throughout life were updated by the U.S. Institutes of Medicine (IOM) in 2010 and are currently set at:

- Infants 0-12 months - 400 IU (10 mcg).
- Children 1-18 years - 600 IU (15 mcg).
- Adults to age 70 - 600 IU (15 mcg).
- Adults over 70 - 800 IU (20 mcg).
- Pregnant or lactating women - 600 IU (15 mcg)

It is estimated that sensible sun exposure on bare skin for 5-10 minutes 2-3 times per week allows most people to produce sufficient vitamin D, but vitamin D breaks down quite quickly, meaning that stores can run low, especially in winter. Although vitamin D supplements can be taken, it is best to obtain any vitamin or mineral through natural sources wherever possible.

Source: https://www.medicalnewstoday.com/articles/161618.php?sr

Part C

In this part of the test, there are two texts about different aspects of healthcare. For **questions 7 to 22**, choose the answer (**A**, **B**, **C** or **D**) which you think fits best according to the text.

Text 1: DNA Testing for Human Papilloma Virus

In Australia, the introduction of the Papanicolaou smear (Pap test) in 1991 has led to the halving of incidence and mortality rates from cervical cancer. Pap smear screening has been delivered through the National Cervical Screening Program (NCSP). The Medical Services Advisory Committee (MSAC) has recently proposed changes to the NCSP to improve its clinical effectiveness and cost-effectiveness. These changes involve replacing the Pap smear with the HPV DNA test as a primary screening tool.

The link between HPV infection and cervical cancer is well established. HPV is spread by genital skin contact during sex. About 4 out of 5 people will be infected with HPV during their lifetime. In most cases, the virus will clear naturally within 1 to 2 years. However, HPV infections that persist for over 3 years are unlikely to be cleared spontaneously and may result in the development of cancerous lesions. This process is dependent upon viral particles gaining access to the epithelial basal layer and entering the dividing cells.

The high-risk genotypes of HPV, those most likely to **_progress_** to intraepithelial lesions, are HPV16, HPV18, HPV45 and HPV31. This is due to the specific activity of their oncogenes. These proteins have a greater ability to drive epithelial cells into the S-phase and continue their replication above the basal layer. The more low-risk genotypes, HPV6 and HPV11, rarely lead to high-grade lesions and are more likely to be associated with genital warts.

The Pap test is the most common screening tool of the current NCSP. It involves sampling cells from the transformational zone with a small spatula or brush. In a liquid-based Pap test, the spatula or brush is immersed in liquid. Under a microscope, the presence of abnormalities in the cells is then assessed. Signs of infection with HPV include the presence of enlarged nuclei with well-defined perinuclear halos, an irregular nuclear membrane and rope-like chromatin (these are called koilocytes). Neoplasia can be identified by the presence of many cells with a high nucleo-cytoplasmic ratio, featuring nuclei with an irregular border.

The current National Cervical Screening Program (NCSP) in Australia uses cytology for screening and histology for diagnosis of cervical cancer. Routine screening is carried out every two years. The screening period begins 1-2 years after first sexual intercourse, or at the age of 18 years, whichever is later. It is recommended until the woman turns 70 years of age.

The results of research studies demonstrate consistently higher sensitivity but lower specificity of HPV DNA testing. This indicates that the HPV DNA test is more accurate than the Pap test in correctly identifying women who have HSIL or cancerous cervical lesions, but less accurate in excluding those who don't. The sensitivity and specificity of HPV DNA testing was more consistently high than that of Pap testing, and specificity increased with age. This indicates that overall, *it* produces more valid results.

There is now robust evidence for the involvement of HPV infection in development of nearly all cases of cervical cancer. Although there are cost-related challenges associated with HPV DNA as a primary screening tool, there are also several ways in which these can be offset. These include better prevention of morbidity and mortality from HPV-related cervical cancer, and aligning the technique with technologies that are already available, such as cytology. Therefore, HPV DNA testing should be employed as the primary screening tool for a revised National Cervical Screening Program, as per the proposal put forward by MSAC.

Text 1: Questions 7 to 14

7. According to the first paragraph, the effect of the Pap smear in Australia has been…
   A   The most effective tool for reducing incidence and mortality from cervical cancer.
   B   A reduction in mortality from cervical cancer to half of the previous rate.
   C   More substantial for incidence than for mortality rates.
   D   Inadequate, so that it is now being replaced with the HPV DNA test.

8. In the second paragraph, the author states that:
   A   The link between HPV and cervical cancer is unclear.
   B   A HPV infection that lasts for 3 or more years will eventually clear by itself.
   C   HPV infection will eventually lead to cervical cancer if untreated.
   D   HPV is unlikely to cause cancerous lesions without entering the epithelial basal layer.

9. The word "***progress***" in the third paragraph could best be replaced with:
   A   Proceed
   B   Promote
   C   Advance
   D   Precede

10. According to the fourth paragraph, the pap test:
    A   Involves taking a biopsy from the transformational zone.
    B   Is the most accurate screening tool for HPV.
    C   Identifies cells with enlarged nuclei.
    D   Requires the assessment of cells under a microscope by a pathologist.

11. The current National Cervical Screening Program recommends:
    A   Cytology and histology of cells for cervical cancer every 2 years.
    B   Routine screening from the age of 18, for the rest of the woman's lifetime.
    C   Commencing screening before the age of 18 for females who become sexually active earlier in life.
    D   2-yearly cytology after a woman's first intercourse or 18th birthday.

12. In the sixth paragraph, "it" refers to:
    A   The pap test.
    B   HPV DNA testing.
    C   Specificity.
    D   Increasing age.

13. In the last paragraph, the author argues that:
- A   HPV DNA testing is superior to the Pap test in all aspects.
- B   The results of HPV DNA testing are more predictable than the Pap test.
- C   The accuracy of HPV DNA testing results make it superior to the Pap test.
- D   The HPV DNA test should be used to exclude high-grade lesions.

14. From the article, it can be argued that:
- A   HPV DNA testing should replace the Pap test in the National Cervical Screening Program.
- B   HPV DNA testing has better accuracy but also significant disadvantages compared to the Pap test.
- C   The National Cervical Screening Program is becoming a more robust health promotion tool in Australia.
- D   There is increasing recognition of cervical cancer being an important public health issue.

Text 2: The Eradication of Smallpox

During the 19th century, the implementation of mandatory, extensive smallpox vaccination led to a substantial decrease in smallpox-related deaths. As early as 1722, James Jurin observed a significant difference between the rates of fatalities in inoculated children (1 in 91) when compared with non-inoculated children (1 in 14). Prior to the widespread use of the vaccine, the fatality rate associated with smallpox usually varied between 20% and 60%. In the infant population this was even higher, with the fatality rate in children under 5 years of age reported to reach up to 80% in London and 98% in Berlin.

As the vaccinated population grew and the incidence of smallpox decreased throughout the world, the development of ***herd immunity*** helped to protect those who could not be immunised. This included very young infants, the very old and the very ill. Mandatory immunisation laws also helped to ensure that disadvantaged children, who would normally be less likely to be vaccinated, received the vaccine.

Although the vaccination process developed by Jenner was relatively safe, there was alarm over a small number of deaths in children after vaccination. There were several serious (although rare) adverse effects reported to the smallpox vaccine as late as the 1960s. In the United States, these included death (1 per million vaccinations), progressive vaccinia (1.5 per million vaccinations), eczema vaccinatum (12 per million vaccinations) and generalised vaccinia (241 per million vaccinations). Inadvertent vaccination, when a person transfers the vaccinia virus from the vaccination site to another part of their body, was the most common adverse event and occurred in 529 vaccinations per million.

Another detrimental outcome related to the mandatory nature of the vaccination itself was the impact on parent-physician relationships. Denying parents the right to refuse the vaccination of their children, except under special circumstances, damages the trust and mutual respect that underpins the relationship between doctors and parents. It is clear that a significant number of parents objected to mandatory smallpox vaccination, and this led to a number of public riots throughout the 19th century.

Despite the rare occurrence of adverse events and lack of universal public acceptance, data from the United Kingdom and Scandinavian countries demonstrate that widespread vaccination of the population against smallpox resulted in a significant decline in smallpox mortality. In turn, this contributed to substantial growth in the European population. The concurrent downward trends In crude death rates and smallpox mortality rates during the first half of the 19th century in Copenhagen, Denmark, provide an interesting view of the impact of the vaccine.

Additionally, data on smallpox mortality rates from Germany and Austria may allow a comparison between the former population, where mandatory vaccination was introduced in 1874 and the latter, where no such measure was taken at that time. In the two decades following the introduction of mandatory vaccination, the mortality rate due to smallpox in Germany rapidly declined, whilst no such decline was observed in Austria. This same pattern of declining mortality from smallpox was seen in other parts of the world, such as the United States.

At the time of Jenner's discovery, the mainstream medical community was skeptical about the value of inoculation as a public health policy. However, as the vaccine's safety and effectiveness improved, so too did its acceptability in the medical community. Today, vaccination is widely used. The practice has made a major contribution to reducing the incidence and burden of many diseases. Although the public debate about vaccination as a health measure continues, it is now regarded as standard medical practice for eligible individuals.

The mandatory nature of vaccination laws also led to a new era in public health surveillance and education. Children were followed up from birth until they had received their vaccination, close contacts of smallpox cases were tracked down and vaccinated, and parents from all social classes made more contact with physicians. The eventual global eradication of smallpox demonstrates the success of this mandatory vaccination policy in disease reduction.

Text 2: Questions 15 to 22

15. According to the first paragraph, the smallpox-related fatality rate of non-inoculated children:
    A   Was different across various European countries.
    B   Was between 20% and 60% prior to the widespread use of the smallpox vaccine.
    C   Was higher than that of inoculated children during the 18th century.
    D   Was as high as 98% in cities such as Berlin.

16. Regarding the concept of "***herd immunity***":
    A   It means that the elderly or very young cannot be immunised against smallpox.
    B   It is necessary in order to achieve complete vaccine coverage within a population.
    C   It is achieved by imposing mandatory vaccination laws.
    D   It involves the vaccinated population protecting the un-vaccinated population from smallpox.

17. In the third paragraph, the adverse effects of smallpox vaccination:
    A   Were rare, but serious enough to attract significant concern.
    B   Included a significant number of deaths.
    C   Only occurred after the administration of 255.5 million vaccinations.
    D   Were isolated to the United States population.

18. Mandatory smallpox vaccination affected parent-physician relationships by:
    A   Denying parents the right to refuse vaccination.
    B   Causing public riots involving parents who objected to mandatory smallpox vaccination.
    C   Underpinning the relationships between parents and doctors.
    D   Undermining the trust and respect that parents have for their child's doctor.

19. The fifth paragraph argues that population growth throughout Europe:
    A   Could not have occurred without a significant decline in smallpox vaccination rates.
    B   Can be attributed to mandatory smallpox vaccination including the UK and Scandinavia.
    C   Was most evident in data from Copenhagen, Denmark.
    D   Was a result of widespread vaccination of the population.

20. According to the sixth paragraph, mandatory vaccination was Introduced:
    A   In Austria in 1874.
    B   In Germany in 1874.
    C   In the European population in 1874.
    D   In the United States.

21. Which of the following best describes the attitude of the medical community towards the smallpox vaccine?

    A   Resistant

    B   Cautious

    C   Embracing

    D   Disapproving

22. One of the main positive outcomes of mandatory smallpox vaccination was:

    A   Children received all their vaccinations from birth onwards.

    B   Close contacts of smallpox cases could be identified and treated.

    C   Parents from all social classes became more comfortable with physicians.

    D   There was increased contact between members of the public and medical doctors.

END OF READING TEST

<h1 style="text-align:center">Test 1: Answer Key</h1>

Part A

Questions 1 to 20

1	B
2	A
3	C
4	C
5	B
6	D
7	A
8	1 to -1
9	to prevent fractures
10	2.07 million **aged over 50**
11	excessive
12	minerals NOT "calcium" only
13	bone health check
14	calcium and vitamin D
15	over 50
16	bone density scan/test
17	vitamin D AND (regular) exercise
18	fragile
19	medical conditions
20	2.07 million

Part B

Questions 1 to 6

1	C	Children receive most of their vaccinations by age 2
2	B	Men should become fertile again once they stop it
3	C	The presence or absence of a person's control over it
4	C	Closely monitor the patient's bowel movements
5	B	Avoid gross contamination of medical devices when possible
6	C	The needs of most adults can be met through adequate sun exposure

Part C

Questions 7 to 14

7	B	A reduction in mortality from cervical cancer to half of the previous rate.
8	D	HPV is unlikely to cause cancerous lesions without entering the epithelial basal layer.
9	C	Advance.
10	C	Identifies cells with enlarged nuclei.
11	D	2-yearly cytology beginning after a woman's first sexual intercourse or her 18th birthday.
12	B	HPV DNA testing.
13	C	The accuracy of HPV DNA testing results make it superior to the Pap test.
14	A	HPV DNA testing should replace the Pap test in the National Cervical Screening Program.

Questions 15 to 22

15	C	Was higher than that of inoculated children during the 18th century.
16	D	It involves the vaccinated population protecting the un-vaccinated population from smallpox.
17	A	Were rare, but serious enough to attract significant concern.
18	D	Undermining the trust and respect that parents have for their child's doctor.
19	B	Can be attributed to mandatory smallpox vaccination including the UK and Scandinavia.
20	B	In Germany in 1874.
21	B	Cautious.
22	D	There was increased contact between members of the public and medical doctors.

END OF KEY

Test 1: Answer Guide

Part A

Text A

Ri: 2 factors for osteoporosis in men
If you have any of the following risk factors, see your doctor for a bone health 13 check:

Personal 19	Medical conditions	Medications	7 Lifestyle issues
Family history	Low testosterone	Treatments for	Smoking
Previous	Coeliac disease	prostate cancer 11	Excessive
fracture	Chronic liver or	Glucocorticoids	alcohol
Loss of height	kidney disease	Anti-epilepsy drugs	Being inactive
(3cm or more)	Rheumatoid	Some anti-	Obesity
	arthritis	depressants	Low body
	Diabetes		weight

Text B

How 1 osteoporosis diagnosed?
Osteoporosis is diagnosed with a bone density scan (i.e. bone density test) 16 result will indicate if bones are in the range of normal, osteopenia or osteoporosis:

T-score	Result	Meaning
1 to -1 8	Normal	17 You should ensure you have adequate calcium, enough Vitamin D and you do regular exercise – these are all important factors for maintaining healthy bones.
-1 to -2.5	Osteopenia 5	Take immediate action to minimize further bone loss. Your doctor will ensure calcium and Vitamin D levels are adequate and discuss any possible risk factors for osteoporosis. Your doctor will monitor your bone density with a follow-up DXA scan after 1-2 years.
-2.5 or lower	Osteoporosis	Your doctor will start treatment with specific osteoporosis medicines and ensure adequate 14 calcium and Vitamin D levels. Follow up tests to monitor bone health.

Text C

FAQs

What is osteoporosis? **4**   **18**

Osteoporosis is a condition in which bones become fragile, leading to a higher risk of fractures (or breaks) than in normal bone. Osteoporosis occurs when bones lose minerals **12** as calcium, more quickly than the body can replace them, leading to a loss of bone thickness (bone mass or density). As a result, bones become thinner and less dense so that even a minor bump or fall can result in a fracture.

Who gets osteoporosis? Can it be treated? **3**

Over 1 million Australians have osteoporosis. It affects both men and women and is most common is adults over 50. Osteoporosis can be treated and there a range of medications available in Australia. It is most important that osteoporosis is detected as early as possible to ensure bone health is managed to prevent fractures.

9

What is a bone density test?

A bone density test is a simple scan that measures the density of your bones (usually at the hip and spine). The results of this test show if your bones are in the range of normal, low bone density or osteoporosis. You doctor will review any risk factors you may have for osteoporosis before referring you for a bone density scan. Medicare rebates apply for many (but not all) cases.

Text D

People in NSW & ACT over 50 estimated to have osteoporosis or osteopenia in 2022

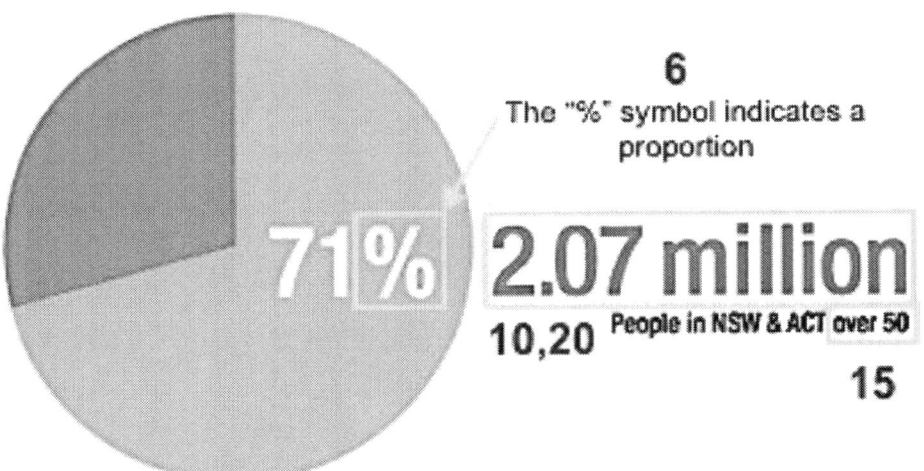

6

The "%" symbol indicates a proportion

71% **2.07 million**

10,20   People in NSW & ACT over 50

15

Part B

1. According to the text
    A   Incorrect: Children are vaccinated against three diseases at one year of age
    B   Incorrect: Children under four years cannot receive the diphtheria vaccination
    C   **Correct: all the vaccinations, expect for those scheduled at 4 years, are given prior to the age of 2.**
2. In terms of male hormonal contraception
    A   Incorrect: This is not referred to in the text.
    B   **Correct: This is the "reversible way" referred to in the text.**
    C   Incorrect: The texts states that progestogen is a synthetic hormone.
3. An addiction can be differentiated from a habit by
    A   Incorrect: Conscious choices are present in both.
    B   Incorrect: Physical signs can be present in both.
    C   **Correct: This is referred to in the first sentence of the text.**
4. Healthcare staff treating patients taking Clozapine should
    A   Incorrect: This is not referred to in the text.
    B   Incorrect: This is not referred to in the text.
    C   **Correct: This is referred to in the text as "close monitoring of bowel function".**
5. Healthcare staff working in operating theatres should
    A   Incorrect: This is not one of the recommendations in the text.
    B   **Correct: This is referred to in the phrase "Keeping instruments free from gross soiling…"**
    C   Incorrect: This refers to "complex and difficult to clean medical devices".
6. Regarding the levels of Vitamin D required
    A   Incorrect: The text states that supplements "can" be taken.
    B   Incorrect: The needs of most adults increase with age, as adults aged over 70 require a larger upper limit (800) than adults to age 70.
    C   **Correct: This is referred to in the phrase "…allows most people to produce sufficient vitamin D".**

Part C

7. According to the first paragraph, the effect of the Pap smear in Australia has been…
    A   Incorrect: The article doesn't compare the Pap smear to other tools that may be used, so we cannot say it is the *most* effective.
    B   **Correct: "the introduction of the Papanicolaou smear (Pap test) in 1991 has led to the halving of incidence and mortality rates from cervical cancer"**
    C   Incorrect: The reductions in incidence and mortality rates are not compared in the article.
    D   Incorrect: The article does not state that the effect of the Pap smear was inadequate.

8. In the second paragraph, the author states that:
   - A Incorrect: "The link between HPV infection and cervical cancer is well established." "Well established" means the opposite of "unclear".
   - B Incorrect: "HPV infections that persist for over 3 years are unlikely to be cleared spontaneously".
   - C Incorrect: "In most cases, the virus will clear naturally within 1 to 2 years."
   - D **Correct: "This process is dependent upon viral particles gaining access to the epithelial basal layer".**

9. The word "***progress***" in the third paragraph could best be replaced with:
   - A Incorrect: the definition of "proceed" is "move forward".
   - B Incorrect: the definition of "promote" is "support or encourage".
   - C **Correct: the definition of "advance" is "make progress".**
   - D Incorrect: the definition of "precede" is "come before".

10. According to the fourth paragraph, the pap test:
   - A Incorrect: the author states that it involves "sampling cells from the transformational zone", but doesn't specifically state that this involves taking a biopsy.
   - B Incorrect: the author states that the pap test is "the most common screening tool", but this doesn't necessarily mean that it is also the most accurate.
   - C **Correct: the test involves assessing for abnormalities, of which "enlarged nuclei with well-defined perinuclear halos" is the first listed.**
   - D Incorrect: this may be true generally, but the article doesn't state who assesses the cells, so we cannot make this conclusion.

11. The current National Cervical Screening Program involves:
   - A Incorrect: "Routine screening is carried out every two years." Since screening refers to cytology, not cytology AND histology, this answer is inaccurate.
   - B Incorrect: Screening is recommended "until the woman turns 70 years of age."
   - C Incorrect: "The screening period begins 1-2 years after first sexual intercourse, or at the age of 18 years, whichever is later." Therefore, if a female becomes sexually active before the age of 18, screening would still not commence until age 18.
   - D **Correct: "The screening period begins 1-2 years after first sexual intercourse, or at the age of 18 years."**

12. In the sixth paragraph, "it" refers to:
   - A Incorrect: This is the test which the subject is compared to.
   - B **Correct: This is the subject of the previous sentence.**
   - C Incorrect: A test, not a particular level of specificity, can be said to produce valid results.
   - D Incorrect: It is a particular test that produces more valid results.

13. In the last paragraph, the author argues that:
   - A Incorrect: The text states that HPV DNA testing is "less accurate in excluding those who don't [have HSIL or cancerous cervical lesions]". Therefore, it isn't superior in all aspects.

B   Incorrect: HPV DNA testing has consistently higher sensitivity and specificity, but this doesn't mean the same as "predictable".

C   Correct: "The sensitivity and specificity of HPV DNA testing was more consistently high than that of Pap testing", meaning that its results are more accurate.

D   Incorrect: The text doesn't explicitly state this. In fact, it states a disadvantage of using HPV DNA testing for this purpose: "less accurate in excluding those who don't [have HSIL or cancerous cervical lesions]".

14. From the article, it can be argued that:

A   **Correct: this view is put forward in the introduction ("The Medical Services Advisory Committee (MSAC) has recently proposed changes to the NCSP to improve its clinical effectiveness and cost-effectiveness. These changes involve replacing the Pap smear with the HPV DNA test") and conclusion ("HPV DNA testing should be employed as the primary screening tool").**

B   Incorrect: The text only mentions one disadvantage of HPV DNA testing (less accuracy in excluding women without HSIL or cancerous cervical lesions), so "significant" is too strong.

C   Incorrect: The text doesn't provide sufficient information about the National Cervical Screening Program to draw this conclusion about the program as a whole. Therefore, this answer is too general.

D   Incorrect: The text doesn't provide any information about the recognition of cervical cancer as a public health issue.

15. According to the first paragraph, the smallpox-related fatality rate of non-inoculated children:

A   Incorrect: The mortality rates for London and Berlin don't provide information specifically about non-inoculated children. They are for all children under 5 years of age.

B   Incorrect: This is the general fatality rate before the smallpox vaccine, not the specific rate for non-inoculated children.

C   Correct: The rate for non-inoculated children was reported to be 1 in 14, which is higher than 1 in 91 (the rate for inoculated children).

D   Incorrect: this is the overall fatality rate for all children under 5 years of age in Berlin, regardless of whether they were inoculated or not.

16. Regarding the concept of herd immunity:

A   Incorrect: This statement is too general. Only some of the elderly or very young may not be able to be immunised.

B   Incorrect: Herd immunity occurs when vaccine coverage is incomplete, but enough people are vaccinated to prevent the spread of a disease.

C   Incorrect: This statement is too broad. Mandatory vaccination is not necessary for herd immunity to occur.

D   Correct: "the development of "herd immunity" helped to protect those who could not be immunised".

17. In the third paragraph, the adverse effects of smallpox vaccination:

A   **Correct: The text states that "there was alarm over a small number of deaths in children after vaccination. There were several serious (although rare) adverse effects..."**

B   Incorrect: The text states that there were "a small number of deaths", which means the opposite to "a significant number".

C   Incorrect: The rates of side effects are given in numbers per million, but the text doesn't state how many vaccines were administered.

D   Incorrect: The rates of adverse effects given are those for the US, but this doesn't mean that they didn't occur in other countries.

18. Mandatory smallpox vaccination affected parent-physician relationships by:

A   Incorrect: The denial of parents' rights to refuse vaccination didn't affect parent-physician relationships directly, but rather, through its effect on trust and respect.

B   Incorrect: The riots didn't directly affect parent-physician relationships.

C   Incorrect: Mandatory vaccination didn't underpin these relationships ("underpin" means "support").

D   **Correct: To undermine means to damage, and the text states that mandatory vaccination denied parents the right to refuse vaccination, which in turn "damages the trust and mutual respect that underpins the relationship between doctors and parents".**

19. The fifth paragraph argues that population growth throughout Europe:

A   Incorrect: The opposite is stated in the text: "widespread vaccination of the population against smallpox resulted in a significant decline in smallpox mortality. In turn, this contributed to substantial growth in the European population."

B   **Correct: The text states: "data from the United Kingdom and Scandinavian countries demonstrate that widespread vaccination of the population against smallpox resulted in a significant decline in smallpox mortality. In turn, this contributed to substantial growth in the European population."**

C   Incorrect: The text states that data from Copenhagen "provide an interesting view of the impact of the vaccine", but this doesn't mean that the impact wasn't clearer in other areas.

D   Incorrect: This is too general. "Widespread smallpox vaccination" would be more accurate.

20. According to the sixth paragraph,

A   Incorrect: This is the population where no such measure was introduced.

B   **Correct: This is the "former (first listed) population" referred to in the text.**

C   Incorrect: This is too general.

D   Incorrect: The introduction of mandatory vaccination in the United States is not referred to in this paragraph.

21. Which of the following best describes the attitude of the medical community towards the smallpox vaccine?

A   Incorrect: This only describes the initial attitude ("skeptical"), which changed as the vaccine's safety and effectiveness improved.

B   **Correct: The medical community was uncertain about the value of the smallpox vaccine until it improved: "as the vaccine's safety and effectiveness improved, so too did its acceptability in the medical community." This describes a cautious approach.**

    C   Incorrect: This is too positive, considering the initial skeptical attitude.

    D   Incorrect: This is implied, but again, only in the initial attitude which later changed.

22. One of the main positive outcomes of mandatory smallpox vaccination was:

    A   Incorrect: "<u>all</u> their vaccinations" is too general, as the article only refers to the smallpox vaccination.

    B   Incorrect: The text states that "close contacts of smallpox cases were tracked down and vaccinated".

    C   Incorrect: The text states that "parents from all social classes made more contact with physicians", but it would be an assumption to state that this means they became more comfortable with physicians.

    D   **Correct: The text states that "parents from all social classes made more contact with physicians".**

56

Test 2

Part A

TIME: 15 minutes

- Look at the four texts, **A – D**, in the separate **Text Booklet**.

- For each question, **1 – 20**, look through the texts, **A – D**, to find the relevant information.

- Write your answers on the spaces provided in this **Question Paper**.

- Answer all the questions within the 15-minute time limit.

Climate Change and Human Health: Questions

Questions 1-7

For each of the questions, **1 – 7**, decide which text (**A**, **B**, **C** or **D**) the information comes from. You may use any letter more than once.

In which text can you find information about

1	How climate change effects are being addressed?	_____
2	Why some people are more affected by climate change?	_____
3	Actions the community can take to address climate change?	_____
4	How climate change can affect our health?	_____
5	Examples of more vulnerable populations?	_____
6	Examples of more sustainable methods of transport?	_____
7	The mechanism of climate-related infections?	_____

Questions 8 – 14

Answer each of the questions, **8 – 14**, with a word or short phrase from one of the texts.

Each answer may include words, numbers or both. Your answers should be correctly spelled.

8   What is one example of an infectious disease altered by climate change?

_____

9   What is a climate-related cause of land loss?

_____

10   How can sustainable transport help the environment?

_____

11   Cutting down on which types of meat might reduce emissions?

_____

12   What is one type of natural event that reduces access to resources?

_____

13   What might conflict zones limit access to?

_____

14   What type of energy might help to mitigate climate change?

_____

58

Questions 15 – 20

Complete each of the sentences, **15 – 20**, with a word or short phrase from one of the texts.
Each answer may include words, numbers or both. Your answers should be correctly spelled.

The groups whose _____ **(15)** can make them more vulnerable to the effects of climate change include ethnic minorities.

Sociopolitical conditions include the presence of _____ **(16)** or conflict.

Altered _____ **(17)** to extreme heat may cause increased morbidity.

The disruption of _____ **(18)** ecosystems may deplete crops and animals.

Some concerning meteorological conditions include _____ **(19)** events.

Shortages of _____ **(20)** will require adaptations in order to be addressed.

Climate Change and Human Health: Texts

Text A

Potential health impacts of climate change
- Milder winters may reduce the peak in winter-time deaths in temperate countries
- Alterations in the geographic range and seasonality of other vector-borne infections, such as malaria and dengue fever
- Increased frequency of diarrhoea in middle-income countries
- Altered patterns of exposure to extreme heat
- Disturbance of natural and food-producing ecosystems, leading to reduced soil fertility and depletion of animals such as ocean fish
- Rising sea levels, leading to population displacement and land loss
- Increased frequency of extreme weather events, such as drought, floods and fires

Source: World Health Organisation

Text B

Current impacts of climate change and responses

Impact pathways		Current responses	
Meteorological conditions exposure	**Human/social consequences of climate change**	**Mitigation actions**	**Adaptation actions**
Examples:	Examples:	Examples:	Examples:
• Warming • Humidity • Rainfall/drying • Winds • Extreme events	• Displacement • Shift in farming and land use	• Alternative energy • Accessible clean water	• Addressing water shortage • Crop substitution • Community education on early warning systems and hazard management

Source: World Health Organisation

60

What makes people vulnerable to the health effects of climate change?	
Vulnerability due to demographic factors:	Proportion of children Proportion of women Proportion of elderly people Population density
Vulnerability due to health status:	Immunocompromised populations Undernourished populations Mentally or physically disabled people
Vulnerability due to culture or life condition:	Impoverished Subsistence farmers and fisher-folk Ethnic minorities Displaced populations
Vulnerability due to limited access to adequate resources/services:	Flood risk zones Drought risk zones Conflict zones Urban, remote, rural areas
Vulnerability due to sociopolitical conditions:	Political instability Existence of complex emergencies or conflict Types of civil rights and civil society

Source: World Health Organisation

Text D

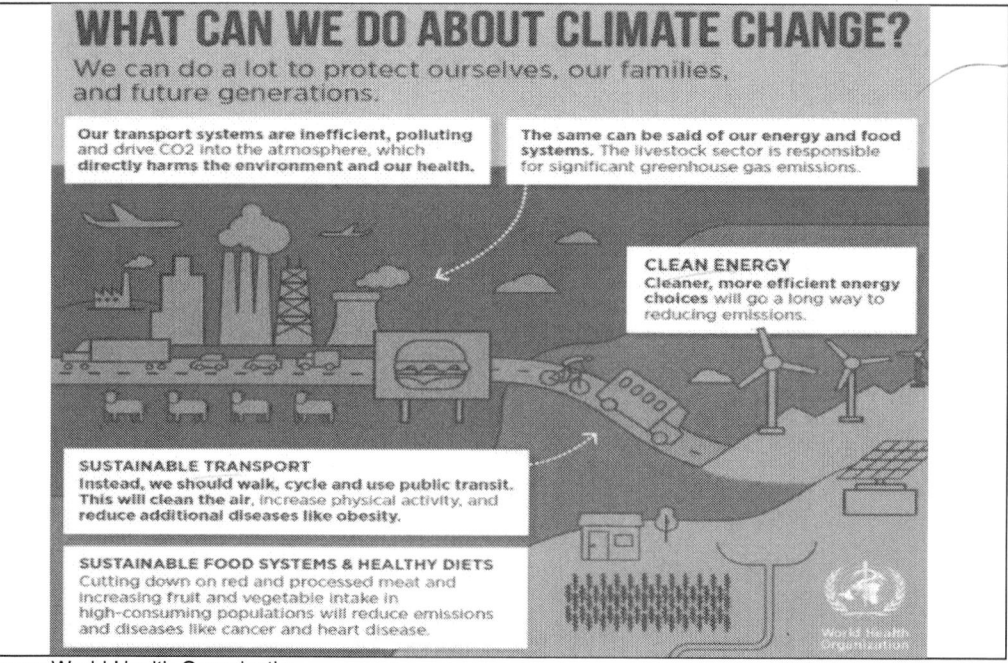

Source: World Health Organisation

END OF PART A
THIS ANSWER BOOKLET WILL BE COLLECTED

Part B

In this part of the test, there are six short extracts relating to the work of health professionals.

For **questions 1 to 6**, choose the answer (**A**, **B** or **C**) which you think fits best according to the text.

---

1. The best conclusion, based on the information in the text, is

    A   Alcohol can both increase and decrease the risk of dementia

    B   Alcohol decreases the risk of dementia with increased consumption

    C   Alcohol and dementia have a dose-response relationship

Some studies have suggested that moderate alcohol intake may have protective effects on the brain, whereas excessive consumption is thought to raise the risk of dementia. However, most of these studies have looked only at alcohol intake in later life, without accounting for the lifetime consumption. Such an approach may have skewed the results. A team of researchers from the French National Institute of Health and Medical Research addressed this by looking at patterns of alcohol consumption from mid-life into old age. Their findings have shown that abstaining from alcohol in midlife and drinking heavily raises the risk of dementia when compared with light-to-moderate drinking. However, the researchers warn, the results of this study "should not motivate people who do not drink to start drinking given the known detrimental effects of alcohol consumption for mortality, neuropsychiatric disorders, cirrhosis of the liver, and cancer."

Source: https://www.medicalnewstoday.com/articles/322659.php

2. A false result will occur when conducting the test below in the case of

    A   The use of urine collected over two days

    B   The use of urine collected over half a day

    C   The use of urine collected from one episode of urination

Test: Urine Free Cortisol	
Specimen:	24-hour urine collection. Incomplete collection will give misleading results.
Method:	Immunoassay.
Reference Interval:	100-300 nmol/24 h
Application:	Diagnosis of adrenocortical hyperfunction as an indicator of adrenocortical activity in the dexamethasone suppression test (long).
Interpretation:	Increased excretion occurs with primary or secondary adrenocortical hyperfunction, although increased levels may also be seen in Obesity, stress, depression and Alcoholism. The test is not used to evaluate adrenal hypofunction. The Synacthen stimulation test is a more appropriate approach in this circumstance.

Source: Arnaldi G et al. *J Clin Endocrinol Metab* 2003; 88(12): 5593-5602

3. The key message conveyed in the charter excerpt below is

    A   Residential care recipients should be treated safely

    B   Residential care recipients should be treated appropriately

    C   Residential care recipients should be treated with respect

---

Care recipients' rights - residential care

Each care recipient has the following rights:

a) to full and effective use of his or her personal, civil, legal and consumer rights;

b) to quality care appropriate to his or her needs;

c) to full information about his or her own state of health and about available treatments;

d) to be treated with dignity and respect, and to live without exploitation, abuse or neglect;

e) to live without discrimination or victimisation, and without being obliged to feel grateful to those providing his or her care and accommodation;

f) to personal privacy;

g) to live in a safe, secure and homelike environment, and to move freely both within and outside the residential care service without undue restriction...*(continued)*

Source: Department of Health. Charter of Care Recipients' Rights and Responsibilities - Residential Care 2018 [Available from: https://agedcare.health.gov.au/publications-and-articles/guides-advice-and-policies/charter-of-care-recipients-rights-and-responsibilities-residential-care.]

4. Mental health professionals should

    A   Be willing to simplify processes and documentation

    B   Be flexible according to the needs of their clients

    C   Be conscious of the needs of intellectually disabled patients

---

In order to best meet the mental health needs of a person with an intellectual disability, mental health professionals must adapt their clinical approach. The key adaptations which will assist the tailoring of mental health consultations are described below.

Preparing for a consultation with a person with an intellectual disability may involve making the following adjustments:

- simplifying appointment and referral letters by using easy English and making reminder phone calls;

- booking an extended consultation to accommodate possible complexity;

- arranging appointments which accommodate the person's preference and facilitate accessibility, such as time, location or any other health considerations;

- preparing for communication needs, for example, ensuring that their preferred communication system is available during the appointment, and where necessary, arranging an interpreter; and

- identifying and accommodating other physical support needs such as those arising from mobility and sensory impairments.

Source: Department of Developmental Disability Neuropsychiatry (2014). Accessible Mental Health Services for People with an Intellectual Disability: A Guide for Providers. Department of Developmental Disability Neuropsychiatry ISBN 978-0-7334-3431-0

5. Based on the guideline below

    A   Stress imaging is superior to exercise stress tests

    B   Stress imaging should be avoided in men

    C   Stress imaging is a desirable testing method for women

---

Exercise stress test in diabetic cardiovascular disease

In asymptomatic patients with diabetes, there is no role for routine stress testing. There is a paucity of data on the predictive power of exercise testing in patients with diabetes, but available data suggest that an ischaemic finding on exercise ECG is predictive of prognosis.

In a study of 1282 patients (15% with diabetes), sensitivity (47% versus 52%) and specificity (81% versus 80%) for exercise treadmill testing were similar in people with and without diabetes.

For patients who can exercise and have resting ECG that is interpretable for ST-segment shifts, exercise ECG is a reasonable option.

Patients who are unable to exercise should undergo a pharmacological stress test with imaging.

Stress imaging studies are superior to exercise stress tests for diagnosis of CAD in women.

Source: Davidson L and Davidson C (2016) BMJ Best Practice: Diabetic Cardiovascular Disease. Updated April 19, 2016.

6. The general idea proposed in the text is

    A   Pre-pregnancy care involves a holistic healthcare approach

    B   Pre-pregnancy care involves monitoring all medical conditions

    C   Pre-pregnancy care involves improved birth outcomes

Every woman aged 15–49 years should be considered for pre-conception care. Pre-conception care is a set of interventions that aim to identify and modify biomedical, behavioural and social risks to a woman's health or pregnancy outcome through prevention and management. This should include smoking cessation and advice to consider abstinence from alcohol (especially in the early stages of pregnancy), folic acid and iodine supplementation, review of immunisation status, medications and chronic medical conditions, especially glucose control in patients with diabetes. There is evidence to demonstrate improved birth outcomes with pre-conception healthcare in women with diabetes, phenylketonuria and nutritional deficiency as well as benefit from the use of folate supplementation and a reduction in maternal anxiety.

Source: Guidelines for preventive activities in general practice, 8th edn. East Melbourne: Royal Australian College of General Practitioners, 2012.

Part C

In this part of the test, there are two texts about different aspects of healthcare. For **questions 7 to 22**, choose the answer (**A**, **B**, **C** or **D**) which you think fits best according to the text.

Text 1: Stigma Associated with Hepatitis C

Hepatitis C, an infection of the liver by the hepatitis C virus (HCV), is an important public health issue both globally and in Australia. Initially the disease is often asymptomatic, but chronically it can lead to cirrhosis of the liver and resultant liver failure, cancer or life-threatening complications such as gastric varices. The burden of disease is expected to rise significantly as those living with chronic Hepatitis C age. Although the disease is curable, less than 2% of those infected are being treated. The disease is highly stigmatised, presenting significant barriers to treatment and important psychological effects.

Strauss & Teixeira (2006) suggest that chronic HCV patients suffer the same experience of discrimination as HIV carriers, stemming from lack of knowledge and prejudice against drug use. Fear of the negative impacts of disclosure is one of the most significant challenges for individuals, compounded by lack of support from the healthcare system. Additionally, those undergoing treatment may be forced to experience social isolation due to side effects. These may persist for up to 6 months, representing an enormous psychosocial cost.

Discrimination by healthcare workers (HCW's) is a well-reported experience. Common reported complaints include lack of follow-up, insensitive disclosure, limited explanation of treatment, short consultations and difficulty accessing services and physicians. This stigma may arise from a lack of knowledge about Hepatitis C among HCW's due to the relatively recent identification of Hepatitis C. As intravenous drug use is a major risk factor, individuals are often treated as persons who 'engage in risky behaviour', inducing shame and lowering self-esteem. This stigma is compounded for those who contracted HCV by other routes such as blood transfusions, who feel unfairly discriminated by the assumption.

Several studies have demonstrated that HCV is perceived to be an inevitable consequence of injecting drugs. Two studies of chronic users raised practicality concerns, quoting that many would choose not to share needles, however, the desire to inject is stronger than the fear of acquiring Hepatitis C. Studies among less frequent injectors presented a cohort that viewed Hepatitis C as a major concern, and associated the diagnosis with the identity of a 'junkie' or 'risky user', adding another dimension to social stigma.

Hepatitis C is viewed to be much less of a threat than HIV, which dominates the concerns of injecting drug users. Hence, HCV treatment is not considered a priority. This belief may be compounded by assumptions made by health professionals - one study compiling accounts of individual's diagnoses reported that health professionals trivialised Hepatitis C in comparison to HIV/AIDS.

Almost all articles reviewed raised concern about the lack of knowledge of the transmission, symptoms, and progression of Hepatitis C, reporting inconsistency in differentiating types of viral hepatitis, acute and chronic hepatitis. This may contribute significantly to ***trivialisation*** of the disease, as much of the chronic stage is often asymptomatic. Another concern repeatedly raised was confusion in interpretation of antibody test results, and deficiencies in adequate follow up procedures by health professionals.

Injecting drug users also face additional treatment considerations. Psychosis and severe depression are important comorbidities found in this population, and contraindicate HCV treatment. Treatment may worsen symptoms, and the accompanying social isolation or instability makes compliance and monitoring extremely difficult. Substance abuse, particularly alcoholism, can worsen the progression of HCV and present a further contraindication to treatment. Furthermore, these comorbidities tend to compound discrimination, cause isolation from social support systems, unemployment and economic instabilities – additional barriers to accessing healthcare.

The increasing prevalence of Hepatitis C and its progressive stages will present an extremely significant burden on Australia's future health system. Considering the size of the public epidemic, and the profound impacts on an individual's physical, social and psychological wellbeing, Hepatitis C has been largely neglected. The discrimination faced by individuals, particularly in the healthcare setting, needs to be addressed to ensure adequate support. The arrival of new treatments has the potential to revolutionise Hepatitis C management and reduce prevalence; however public health strategies need to be improved to specifically target barriers faced by the injection drug using population in order to reduce incidence.

Text 1: Questions 7 to 14

7. According to the first paragraph,
    A   Hepatitis C is the primary cause of liver failure, cancer and cirrhosis in Australia.
    B   Less than 2% of people with Hepatitis C require treatment.
    C   The stigma associated with Hepatitis C leads to stress and reduced access to treatment.
    D   Most cases of Hepatitis C are asymptomatic.

8. According to Strauss & Teixeira, the experience of HCV patients:
    A   Is the same as that of HIV patients.
    B   Is partially due to ignorance and popular attitudes towards drug users.
    C   Is a significant challenge for individuals within the health system.
    D   Involves social isolation, leading to psychosocial consequences.

9. Regarding discrimination by healthcare workers, which of the following is LEAST correct?
    A   HCV patients often receive inadequate time and empathy from health care workers.
    B   Treatment options following a diagnosis are often insufficiently discussed.
    C   The attitudes of healthcare workers often cause HCV patients to feel worse about themselves.
    D   Healthcare workers often assume that patients with HCV used drugs, regardless of the route of transmission.

10. Which of the following would best summarise the fourth paragraph?
    A   According to drug users, Hepatitis C is a natural consequence of risky injection practices.
    B   Intravenous drug users see Hepatitis C as a major concern.
    C   The desire to inject drugs can overpower safety concerns.
    D   Injection drug users strongly discourage people from getting involved in the practice.

11. Compared to HIV, Hepatitis C:
    A   Is viewed to be less of a problem.
    B   Is believed to be easier to treat.
    C   Is less concerning to healthcare professionals.
    D   Is less likely to lead to AIDS.

12. Which of these could best replace the word "***trivialisation***" in the sixth paragraph?
    A   Misdiagnosis
    B   Underestimation
    C   Ignorance
    D   Stigmatisation

70

13. Regarding the comorbidities described in the seventh paragraph, why are psychosis and depression important?

    A The treatments for these conditions have interactions with the treatments for HCV.

    B They lead to social isolation and instability amongst infected injection drug users.

    C They can lead to substance abuse, which can cause HCV to progress more rapidly.

    D Treating HCV may worsen the symptoms of these conditions, reducing HCV treatment compliance.

14. According to the article, which statement best represents the author's opinion?

    A Hepatitis C is becoming an increasingly significant public health problem in Australia.

    B The stigma faced by people with Hepatitis C deserves greater attention from the healthcare sector.

    C Injecting drug users with Hepatitis C face significant barriers to successful treatment.

    D Hepatitis C is often underestimated due to a fear of other diseases such as HIV.

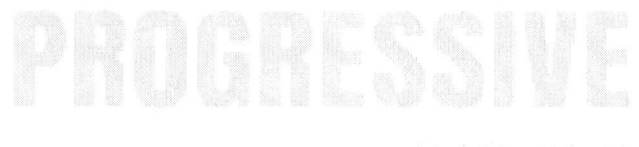

Text 2: The Impact of Household Air Pollution on Health

Household air pollution from biomass fuels used for cooking and heating contributes significantly to global burden of respiratory disease, and disproportionately affects low and middle income countries. Inhalation of toxic pollutants elevates risk of respiratory conditions, particularly acute lower respiratory infections in children and chronic obstructive pulmonary disease (COPD) in women. Women and children in developing countries are most vulnerable due to increased time spent indoors. Public health interventions such as improved cooking stoves and use of cleaner fuels may help reduce mortality and morbidity caused by household air pollution.

Approximately 3 billion people, or 50% of the world's population, rely on solid fuels for domestic cooking and heating. Biomass fuels are used in low and middle income countries due to limited access to cleaner fuels. Worldwide, 3.5 – 4 million deaths are caused by household air pollution annually. Household air pollution is the biggest environmental risk factor, responsible for 3.3% of annual mortality and 2.7% of Disability Adjusted Life Years. Pneumonia and COPD account for 12% and 22% of mortality respectively. The remainder is mostly due to stroke, ischemic heart disease, and lung cancer.

In developing countries, lower respiratory infections such as pneumonia are the leading cause of mortality in children under 5, with over 1.3 million deaths annually. Over 50% of premature deaths in this age group are due to household air pollution-related pneumonia. Children exposed to household air pollution have approximately twice the risk of developing pneumonia, according to meta-analysis (OR 1.78, 95% CI). COPD includes a range of clinical conditions such as emphysema and chronic bronchitis, and is the third leading cause of mortality worldwide. In low and middle income countries, household air pollution is responsible for 35% of COPD prevalence and one third of premature deaths from COPD. Women exposed to household air pollution are at 2 – 3 times greater risk of developing COPD, especially those in rural areas.

Combustion of biomass fuels produces high concentrations of toxic pollutants, including carbon monoxide and particulate matter (PM). Chronic household air pollution exposure leads to inflammation, oxidative stress and DNA damage. Host immune defenses are impaired due to damage to respiratory epithelium by toxic particle deposits, including loss of epithelial integrity, reduced mucociliary function and impaired alveolar macrophage phagocytosis. This increases susceptibility to bacterial invasion and thus acute lower respiratory infections such as pneumonia. Risk of COPD is also increased with chronic household air pollution exposure, comparable to long-term tobacco smoking in clinical presentation and prognosis. Household air pollution can thus cause irreversible damage to respiratory function.

Women and children in poverty are most vulnerable to respiratory diseases caused by household air pollution. This is due to greater time spent indoors and exposure to highest concentrations of toxic pollutants. Culturally, women and girls are more involved in cooking than men. Young children in close proximity to mothers during these times are also heavily exposed to cooking smoke, such as infants carried on the back or laid nearby to sleep. Typically, household air pollution-associated COPD affects "elderly women with life-long exposure from solid fuel use". In addition, hours spent every day gathering fuel amongst other domestic duties limits women and children's productive time to pursue income generation or education.

Poverty is the biggest factor influencing biomass fuel use. Cheaper fuels that produce more pollutants are used in households with lower incomes and poorly **_ventilated_** homes. Cleaner energy such as electricity or liquefied petroleum gas (LPG) is unaffordable, whereas charcoal, wood, dung and crop residues are cheaper. These cheaper fuels have poorer combustion efficiency and produce more smoke/pollutants.

Fuel availability also influences household biomass use and accounts for different fuel use worldwide. Wood is commonly used in India and parts of Africa; coal in China; animal dung in rural/pastoralist communities across Nepal and African savannah regions. Lack of transport or reliable supply limits access to cleaner fuels in rural/resource-poor communities. These difficulties force households to revert to cheaper, more readily available biomass fuels, even after temporary adoption of cleaner fuels.

Worldwide, 3 billion people rely on biomass fuels for domestic purposes, increasing exposure to toxic pollutants endangering their health. Household air pollution is a major risk factor for respiratory disease amongst women and children in developing countries. Improved cooking stoves and cleaner fuel use offer promising solutions to the dilemma of household air pollution-related respiratory diseases, however, addressing household needs and local community involvement are necessary for these interventions to be effective and long-lasting.

Text 2: Questions 15 to 22

15. Respiratory disease due to household air pollution…
    A Is the main side effect of cooking with biomass fuel.
    B Increases the risk of acute lower respiratory infections in women and children.
    C Is more likely to develop in those who spend more time indoors.
    D Only affects women and children in low and middle income countries.

16. From the statistics in the second paragraph, it can be inferred that:
    A Low and middle income countries have a collective population of approximately 3 billion.
    B Residents of high income countries have sufficient access to cleaner fuels.
    C Household air pollution is more likely to cause death than disability.
    D Respiratory diseases account for over a third of deaths related to household air pollution.

17. According to the third paragraph,
    A Lower respiratory tract infections are the leading cause of death in children.
    B Most of the premature deaths in children aged under 5 are due to pneumonia.
    C COPD is a common cause of conditions such as emphysema and bronchitis.
    D Household air pollution causes 35% of COPD prevalence around the world.

18. Toxic pollutants cause respiratory tract damage by:
    A Weakening the immune system's ability to protect and repair the respiratory lining.
    B Carrying bacteria into the lower respiratory tract and causing chronic infection.
    C Making inhabitants who use biomass fuels more likely to start tobacco smoking.
    D Damaging alveolar macrophages, thus preventing phagocytosis.

19. According to the fifth paragraph, infants are affected by household air pollution because:
    A Cultural expectations mean that children are more involved in cooking than men.
    B They have an immature respiratory system that is more susceptible to toxins.
    C They are carried by their mothers, who are involved in most of the cooking.
    D They spend the greatest amount of time indoors.

20. Which of the following would best replace the word "***ventilated***" in the sixth paragraph?
  A Oxygenated
  B Designed
  C Accessed
  D Equipped

21. What is the main impact of fuel availability on household use?
  A Deficiencies in transport and unreliable supply lead to limited access.
  B Rural or resource-poor households are forced to use fuels with more toxic pollutants.
  C Wood and animal dung have become the primary source of cooking fuel.
  D Animal dung is used throughout Nepal and African savannah regions.

22. Regarding the solutions to household air pollution, what does the author suggest?
  A That it is a major risk factor for respiratory disease in women and children.
  B That improved cooking stoves and cleaner fuel use are appropriate solutions.
  C That interventions which aren't community-oriented are unlikely to succeed.
  D That household incomes must be increased before the problem can be solved.

Test 2: Answer Key

Part A

Questions 1 to 20

1	B
2	C
3	D
4	A
5	C
6	D
7	A
8	malaria OR dengue fever
9	rising sea levels
10	clean the air
11	red and processed
12	flood OR drought
13	resources OR services
14	alternative
15	culture or life condition
16	complex emergencies
17	patterns of exposure
18	natural and food-producing
19	extreme
20	water

Part B

Questions 1 to 6

1	A	Alcohol can both increase and decrease the risk of dementia
2	B	The use of urine collected over half a day
3	B	Residential care recipients should be treated appropriately
4	B	Be flexible according to the needs of their clients
5	C	Stress imaging is a desirable testing method for women
6	A	Pre-pregnancy care involves a holistic healthcare approach

Part C

Questions 7 to 14

7	C	The stigma associated with Hepatitis C leads to stress and reduced access to treatment.
8	B	Is partially due to ignorance and popular attitudes towards drug users.
9	D	Healthcare workers often assume that patients with HCV used drugs, regardless of the route of transmission.
10	A	According to drug users, Hepatitis C is a natural consequence of risky injection practices.
11	A	Is viewed to be less of a problem.
12	B	Underestimation
13	D	Treating HCV may worsen the symptoms of these conditions, reducing HCV treatment compliance.
14	B	The stigma faced by people with Hepatitis C deserves greater attention from the healthcare sector.

Questions 15 to 22

15	C	Is more likely to develop in those who spend more time indoors.
16	D	Respiratory diseases account for over a third of deaths related to household air pollution.
17	B	Most of the premature deaths in children aged under 5 are due to pneumonia.
18	A	Weakening the immune system's ability to protect and repair the respiratory lining.
19	C	They are carried by their mothers, who are involved in most of the cooking.
20	A	Oxygenated.
21	B	Rural or resource-poor households are forced to use fuels with more toxic pollutants.
22	C	That interventions which aren't community-oriented are unlikely to succeed.

END OF KEY

Test 2: Answer Guide

Part A

Potent 4 health impacts of climate change
- Mild..r winters may reduce the peak in winter-time deaths in temperate countries
- Alterations in the geographic range and seasonality of other vector-borne infections, such as malaria and dengue fever **7,8**
- Increased frequency of diarrhoea in middle-income countries
17 Altered patterns of exposure to extreme heat
- Disturban **18** natural and food-producing ecosystems, leading to reduced soil fertility and depletion of animals such as ocean fish
9 Rising sea levels, leading to population displacement and land loss
- Increased frequency of extreme weather events, such as drought, floods and fires

Current impacts of climate change a 1 responses

Impact pathways		Current responses	
Meteorological conditions exposure	Human/social consequences of climate change	Mitigation actions	Adaptation actions
Examples:	*Examples:*	*Examples:*	*Examples:*
• Warming	• Displacement	**14** • Alternative energy	**20** Addressing water shortage
• Humidity	• Shift in farming and land use	• Accessible clean water	• Crop substitution
• Rainfall/drying			• Community education on early warning systems and hazard management
• Winds			
• Extreme events **19**			

Text C

What makes people vulnerable 2,5 ? health effects of climate change?	
Vulnerability due to demographic factors:	Proportion of children Proportion of women Proportion of elderly people Population density
Vulnerability due to health status:	Immunocompromised populations Undernourished populations Mentally or physically disabled people
Vulnerability due to culture or life condition: 15	Impoverished Subsistence farmers and fisher-folk Ethnic minorities Displaced populations
Vulnerability due to limited access to adequate resources/services: 13	Flood risk zones 12 Drought risk zones Conflict zones Urban, remote, rural areas
Vulnerability due to sociopolitical conditions:	Political instability Existenc 16 complex emergencies or conflict Types of civil rights and civil society

Text D

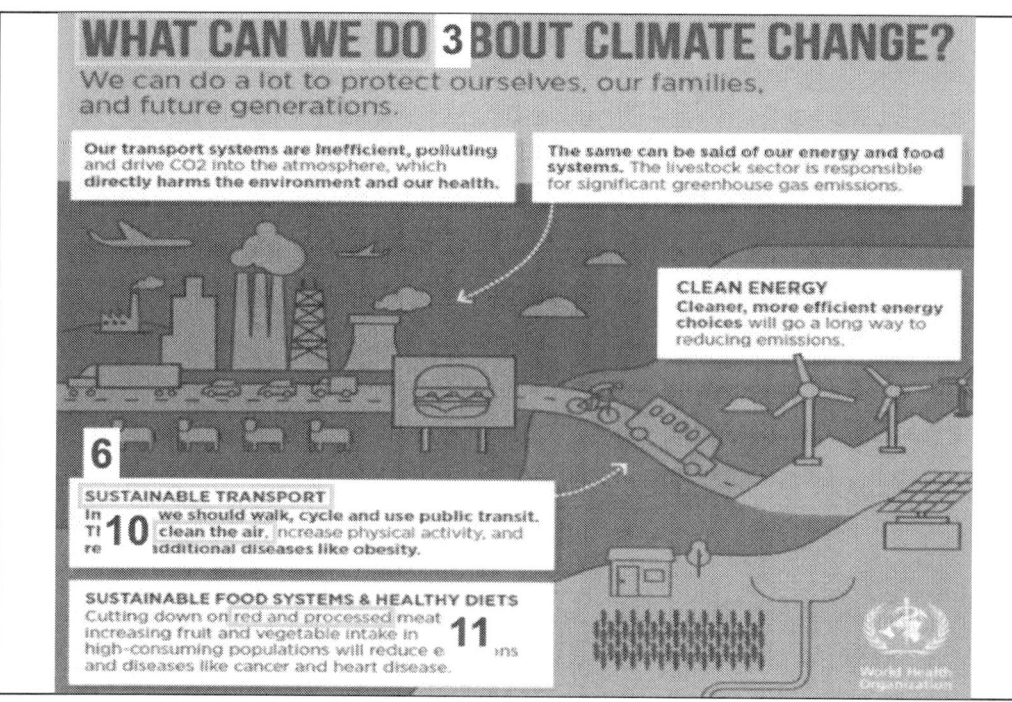

Part B

1. The best conclusion, based on the information in the text, is
    - A **Correct: The text states that "abstaining...AND drinking heavily raises the risk of dementia.**
    - B Incorrect: The text states that "drinking heavily raises the risk of dementia", so this cannot always be true.
    - C Incorrect: This would mean that reducing the amount of alcohol consumed would decrease the risk of dementia, but since abstaining (not drinking) "raises the risk of dementia", this cannot be correct.
2. A false result will occur when conducting the test below in the case of
    - A Incorrect: For example, the 24-hour period may go from 9am on Monday to 9am on Tuesday, which means it would be "over two days".
    - B **Correct: This would provide insufficient urine, as it is less than 24 hours.**
    - C Incorrect: If this is the only urine passed over 24 hours, then this shouldn't cause a false result.
3. The key message conveyed in the charter excerpt below is
    - A Incorrect: This is a minor point, so it is not the key (main) message.
    - B **Correct: The term "appropriately" can be a synonym for referring to all the rights listed in the text.**
    - C Incorrect: This is only one point in the text, so it is not the key (main) message.
4. Mental health professionals should
    - A Incorrect: This is a minor point in the text, so it is not the best answer.
    - B **Correct: This answer encompasses answers A and C, as well as other recommended actions (preparing for communication needs, identifying and accommodating, etc), so it is the best answer.**
    - C Incorrect: This is a minor point in the text, so it is not the best answer.
5. Based on the guideline below
    - A Incorrect: This is only the case for women according to the text, so this answer is too general.
    - B Incorrect: This is not stated or implied in the text.
    - C **Correct: This is stated in the phrase "superior to exercise stress tests...in women".**
6. The general idea proposed in the text is
    - A **Correct: This is a good summary of the points in the text, which refer to addressing multidimensional (holistic) aspects of the woman's health.**
    - B Incorrect: This is a minor point, so it is not the best answer.
    - C Incorrect: This is a minor point, so it is not the best answer.

Part C

7. According to the first paragraph,
    A Incorrect: Although the text states that Hepatitis C "can lead to cirrhosis of the liver and resultant liver failure, cancer or life-threatening complications such as gastric varices", this doesn't mean it is the primary cause.
    B Incorrect: The text states that "less than 2% of those infected are being treated".
    C **Correct: The text states "The disease is highly stigmatised, presenting significant barriers to treatment ("reduced access to treatment") and important psychological effects ("stress")."**
    D Incorrect: The text states that "Initially the disease is often asymptomatic", but not that most cases remain this way.

8. According to Strauss & Teixeira, the experience of HCV patients:
    A Incorrect: The text only states this in reference to their experience of discrimination: "HCV patients suffer the same experience *of discrimination* as HIV carriers..."
    B **Correct: The text states that the experience of discrimination is "stemming from lack of knowledge ("ignorance") and prejudice ("popular attitudes") against drug use."**
    C Incorrect: The text states that it is a significant challenge for individuals "compounded by lack of support from the healthcare system".
    D Incorrect: The text only states this in relation to HCV patients undergoing treatment: "those undergoing treatment may be forced to experience social isolation". Hence, this answer is to general.

9. Regarding discrimination by healthcare workers, which of the following is LEAST correct?
    A Incorrect: In the text, this is referred to by the words "lack of follow-up" and "short consultations" ("inadequate time") and "insensitive disclosure" ("inadequate empathy"). Therefore, it is not the correct choice.
    B Incorrect: In the text, this is referred to by the words "limited explanation of treatment". Therefore, it is not the correct choice.
    C Incorrect: In the text, this is referred to in the statement "individuals are often treated as persons who 'engage in risky behaviour', inducing shame and lowering self-esteem." Therefore, it is not the correct choice.
    D **Correct: The text does state that "This stigma is compounded for those who contracted HCV by other routes such as blood transfusions, who feel unfairly discriminated by the assumption" but it does NOT say that this happens "often", as in the answer. Therefore, this is the correct choice.**

10. Which of the following would best summarise the fourth paragraph?
    A **Correct: This option refers to the topic sentence, supporting information and concluding sentence of the paragraph, so it is a good summary.**
    B Incorrect: This is a minor point in the paragraph, so it doesn't provide a good summary.

C Incorrect: This is a minor point in the paragraph, so it doesn't provide a good summary.

D Incorrect: The message that injecting drug users for other people isn't mentioned in the paragraph.

11. Compared to HIV, Hepatitis C:

    A **Correct: This is referred to in the text by the statement "HIV...dominates the concerns of injecting drug users. Hence, HCV treatment is not considered a priority." (paragraph 5)**

    B Incorrect: Although the text states that "HCV treatment is not considered a *priority*", this doesn't mean that it is *easy* to treat.

    C Incorrect: This is not mentioned in the text.

    D Incorrect: This is not mentioned in the text.

12. Which of these could best replace the word "*trivialisation*" in the sixth paragraph?

    A Incorrect: The definition of "misdiagnosis" is an incorrect diagnosis of an illness or other problem.

    B **Correct: The definition of "trivialisation" is an act of making something seem less significant than it really is.**

    C Incorrect: The definition of "ignorance" is lack of knowledge/information.

    D Incorrect: The definition of "stigmatisation" is the unfair treatment of someone through disapproval.

13. Regarding the comorbidities described in the seventh paragraph, why are psychosis and depression important?

    A Incorrect: The text doesn't mention any treatment interactions.

    B Incorrect: The text does state this, but this is not the main reason why these conditions are important.

    C Incorrect: The text doesn't state that these conditions may lead to substance abuse.

    D **Correct: The text states "*Treatment may worsen symptoms*, and the accompanying social isolation or instability makes *compliance and monitoring extremely difficult*".**

14. According to the article, which statement best represents the author's opinion?

    A Incorrect: This is only mentioned in the introduction.

    B **Correct: This is the main opinion put forward by the author. Examples of where this is expressed are found in the introduction ("The disease is highly stigmatised, presenting significant barriers to treatment and important psychological effects.") and conclusion ("discrimination faced by individuals, particularly in the healthcare setting, needs to be addressed" and "public health strategies need to be improved to specifically target barriers").**

    C Incorrect: This is a fact, not an opinion.

    D Incorrect: This is a fact, and only mentioned at one point in the article, so it is not a main idea.

15. Respiratory disease due to household air pollution...

    A Incorrect: The text states that "Household air pollution from biomass fuels...contributes significantly to global burden of respiratory disease" but doesn't state that this is the *main* side effect.

    B Incorrect: The text only states this for children, not for women.

    C **Correct: The text states that "Women and children in developing countries are most vulnerable *due to increased time spent indoors*".**

    D Incorrect: The text states that "Women and children in developing countries are *most* vulnerable", but not that they are the only ones affected.

16. From the statistics in the second paragraph, it can be inferred that:

    A Incorrect: The text states that "3 billion people, or 50% of the world's population, rely on solid fuels for domestic cooking and heating" but not that all of these people are in low or middle income countries.

    B Incorrect: This is an assumption, as the text doesn't mention this population's access to cleaner fuels.

    C Incorrect: The text states that household air pollution is "responsible for 3.3% of annual mortality and 2.7% of Disability Adjusted Life Years" but the actual size of these proportions in number of people affected is not given.

    D **Correct: The text states that "Pneumonia and COPD account for 12% and 22% of mortality respectively". This adds up to 34%, which is just over a third.**

17. According to the third paragraph,

    A Incorrect: The text states that "lower respiratory infections...are the leading cause of mortality in children *under 5*", so this is too general.

    B **Correct: The text states that "Over 50% (*most*) of premature deaths in this age group are due to household air pollution-related pneumonia."**

    C Incorrect: Emphysema and bronchitis are examples of COPD, not consequences of it ("COPD includes a range of clinical conditions such as emphysema and chronic bronchitis").

    D Incorrect: This is only stated for "low and middle income countries", so this answer is too broad.

18. Toxic pollutants cause respiratory tract damage by:

    A **Correct: This is stated in the text: "Host immune defenses are impaired...loss of epithelial integrity, reduced mucociliary function and impaired alveolar macrophage phagocytosis."**

    B Incorrect: The pollutant "increases susceptibility to bacterial invasion" but doesn't actively carry bacteria itself.

    C Incorrect: The text only states that the risk of COPD is "comparable to long-term tobacco smoking".

    D Incorrect: The text states that there is "impaired alveolar macrophage phagocytosis" but this doesn't necessarily mean that the macrophages themselves are damaged.

19. According to the fifth paragraph, infants are affected by household air pollution because:

    A Incorrect: The text only states that "women and girls are more involved in cooking than men", whereas "children" includes both girls and boys.

    B Incorrect: The child's immune system isn't discussed.

C **Correct: This is stated in the text: "Young children in close proximity to mothers during these times are also heavily exposed to household air pollution, such as infants carried on the back".**

D Incorrect: The text does state that children have a "greater time spent indoors", but this has a slightly different meaning to "greatest".

20. Which of the following would best replace the word "*__ventilated__*" in the sixth paragraph?

A **Correct: "Oxygenated" and "ventilated" both mean having air enter and circulate freely.**

B Incorrect: "Designed" is too general in its meaning.

C Incorrect: "Accessed" is too general in its meaning.

D Incorrect: "Equipped" is too general in its meaning.

21. What is the main impact of fuel availability on household use?

A Incorrect: The text states that this "limits access to *cleaner fuels in rural/resource-poor communities*", so the answer is too broad.

B **Correct: This answer is from the last two sentences of the paragraph: "Lack of transport or reliable supply limits access to cleaner fuels in rural/resource-poor communities. These difficulties force households to revert to cheaper, more readily available biomass fuels"**

C Incorrect: Both fuels are commonly used is certain areas, but this doesn't mean that they are the primary fuel used.

D Incorrect: The text is more specific than this: animal dung is used "in *rural/pastoralist communities* across Nepal and African savannah regions".

22. Regarding the solutions to household air pollution, what does the author suggest?

A Incorrect: This isn't a suggestion about solutions to household air pollution, so it doesn't answer the question.

B Incorrect: This is inaccurate, since the text states that "addressing household needs and local community involvement are necessary for these interventions to be effective and long-lasting."

C **Correct: This is implied in the author's statement: "local community involvement is necessary for these interventions to be effective".**

D Incorrect: The increasing of household incomes isn't suggested by the author as a solution in itself.

Test 3

Part A

TIME: 15 minutes

- Look at the four texts, **A – D**, in the separate **Text Booklet**.

- For each question, **1 – 20**, look through the texts, **A – D**, to find the relevant information.

- Write your answers on the spaces provided in this **Question Paper**.

- Answer all the questions within the 15-minute time limit.

Oral Rehydration Therapy: Questions

Questions 1-7

For each of the questions, **1 – 7**, decide which text (**A**, **B**, **C** or **D**) the information comes from. You may use any letter more than once.

In which text can you find information about

1   The ingredients found in oral rehydration salts?   _____

2   Research on how we can treat cholera?   _____

3   How oral rehydration salts work?   _____

4   The effects of diarrhoea on the body?   _____

5   How citrate helps the body?   _____

6   How dehydration can be prevented?   _____

7   Why diarrhoea requires sodium replacement?   _____

Questions 8 – 14

Answer each of the questions, **8 – 14**, with a word or short phrase from one of the texts.

Each answer may include words, numbers or both. Your answers should be correctly spelled.

8   Which component of ORS has the fewest grams per liter?

_____

9   How was the oral solution administered in the study by Pierce et al?

_____

10   In the same study, what did one patient require small amounts of?

_____

11   Acute diarrhoeal diseases are a leading cause of death in which groups?

_____

12   Who can deliver oral rehydration therapy for diarrhoea?

_____

13   Where is the glucose found in ORS absorbed?

_____

14   How long can ORS be stored for safely?

_____

Questions 15 – 20

Complete each of the sentences, **15 – 20**, with a word or short phrase from one of the texts.
Each answer may include words, numbers or both. Your answers should be correctly spelled.

Adding citrate to ORS makes it particularly useful in _____ **(15)** where temperatures can be quite high.

The duration of diarrhoea was _____ **(16)** in the study by Pierce et al.

Researchers observed a _____ **(17)** increased in stool output amongst some patients.

The main component of the new ORS formulation is _____ **(18)**.

The World Health Organisation recommends that ORT is _____ **(19)** advice on food intake.

The ease of administration of ORT makes it _____ **(20)** to a home or village environment.

Oral Rehydration Therapy: Texts

Text A

Diarrhoea and Oral Rehydration Therapy
Acute diarrhoeal diseases are one of the leading causes of mortality in infants and young children in many developing countries. In most cases, death is caused by dehydration.
Dehydration from diarrhoea can be prevented by giving extra fluids at home, or it can be treated simply, effectively, and cheaply in all age-groups and in all but the most severe cases by giving patients by mouth an adequate glucose-electrolyte solution.
This way of giving fluids to prevent or treat dehydration is called oral rehydration therapy (ORT). ORT, combined with guidance on appropriate feeding practices, is the main strategy recommended by the WHO Department of Child and Adolescent Health and Development (CAH) to achieve a reduction in diarrhoea-related mortality and malnutrition in children.
Oral rehydration therapy (ORT) can be delivered by village health workers and practiced in the home by mothers with some guidance, and thus is a technology highly suited to the primary health care approach.

Source: World Health Organisation

Text B

TABLE 1. Composition of the new ORS formulation

New ORS	grams/litre	%	New ORS	mmol/litre
Sodium chloride	2.6	12.683	Sodium	75
Glucose, anhydrous	13.5	65.854	Chloride	65
Potassium chloride	1.5	7.317	Glucose, anhydrous	75
Trisodium citrate, dihydrate	2.9	14.146	Potassium	20
			Citrate	10
Total	**20.5**	**100.00**	**Total Osmolarity**	**245**

Source: World Health Organisation

88

Abstract: Replacement of Water and Electrolyte Losses in Cholera by an Oral Glucose-Electrolyte Solution (Pierce et al, 1969)

Background: The efficacy of an orally administered glucose-electrolyte solution in replacing stool losses of water and electrolytes in severe cholera was evaluated.

Methods: After initial intravenous rehydration, intravenous fluids were discontinued, and subsequent water and electrolyte losses were replaced by the oral solution administered via nasogastric tube.

Results: In 9 of 10 patients so treated, water, electrolyte, and acid-base balances were adequately maintained by this method until diarrhoea ended. One patient with very severe diarrhoea required small amounts of additional intravenous fluids to maintain water balance. Patients receiving the oral solution had a small but significant increase in stool output during oral fluid administration when compared with the 10 patients in the control group who received only intravenous replacement of stool losses. Calculated absorption of the oral fluid was 87%.

Conclusion: Duration of diarrhoea and of VIBRIO CHOLERAE excretion were not prolonged by the oral solution administration. The role of glucose in the absorption of water and sodium by the small bowel is discussed. The study suggests a useful role for such an orally administered glucose-electrolyte solution in the management of cholera.

Source: Pierce NF, Sack RB, Mitra RC, Banwell JG, Brigham KL, Fedson DS, et al. Replacement of Water and Electrolyte Losses in Cholera by an Oral Glucose—Electrolyte Solution. Ann Intern Med. 1969;70:1173–1181

Therapeutic Mechanisms of ORS

The pharmacokinetics and mechanisms of therapeutic action of the substances in the ORS solution are as follows:

- Glucose facilitates the absorption of sodium (and hence water) on a 1:1 molar basis in the small intestine.
- Sodium and potassium are needed to replace the body losses of these essential ions during diarrhoea (and vomiting).
- Citrate corrects the acidosis that occurs as a result of diarrhoea and dehydration. The particular advantage of citrate containing ORS (over bicarbonate containing ORS) is its stability in tropical countries where temperatures up to 60°C can occur. A shelf-life of 2-3 years can be assumed without any particular storage precautions.

Source: World Health Organisation

END OF PART A
THIS ANSWER BOOKLET WILL BE COLLECTED

Part B

In this part of the test, there are six short extracts relating to the work of health professionals.

For **questions 1 to 6**, choose the answer (**A**, **B** or **C**) which you think fits best according to the text.

---

1. Healthcare workers who are in a teaching position should

     A   Make sure patients maintain their own comfort and dignity

     B   Put patient care above their students' educational needs

     C   Make sure patients are fully informed of the student's role

Code of Ethics: Clinical Teaching

- Honour your obligation to pass on your professional knowledge and skills to colleagues and students.

- Before embarking on any clinical teaching involving patients, ensure that patients are fully informed and have consented to participate.

- Respect the patient's right to refuse or withdraw from participating in clinical teaching at any time without compromising the doctor-patient relationship or appropriate treatment and care.

- Avoid compromising patient care in any teaching exercise. Ensure that your patient is managed according to the best-proven diagnostic and therapeutic methods and that your patient's comfort and dignity are maintained at all times.

- Where relevant to clinical care, ensure that it is the treating doctor who imparts feedback to the patient.

- Refrain from exploiting students or colleagues under your supervision in any way.

Source: Australian Medical Association (2006) AMA Code of Ethics.

2. The grading system below aims to

    A   Identify the ability of the patient to perform daily functions

    B   Identify the greatest level of functioning for the patient being tested

    C   Identify the greatest level of disability for the patient being tested

---

Limb Strength

The weakest muscle in each group defines the score for that muscle group. Use of functional tests, such as hopping on one foot and walking on heels / toes, are recommended in order to assess BMRC grades 3–5.

0 = no muscle contraction detected

1 = visible contraction without visible joint movement

2 = visible movement only on the plane of gravity

3 = active movement against gravity, but not against resistance

4 = active movement against resistance, but not full strength

5 = normal strength

Functional Tests

Pronator Drift (upper extremities):

0 = none

1 = mild

2 = evident

Position Test (lower extremities – ask patient to lift both legs together, with legs fully extended at the knee). Assess whether sinking is:

0 = none

1 = mild

2 = evident

3 = able to lift only one leg at a time

4 = unable to lift one leg at a time

Source: Kurtzke, JF (2009) Definitions for a standardised, quantified neurological examination and assessment of Kurtzke's Functional Systems and Expanded Disability Status Scale in Multiple Sclerosis. Neurology 1983:33,1444-52

3. Patient-reported outcomes

    A   Can often be surprising to their treating clinicians

    B   Are sometimes very different to the actual stage of their condition

    C   Closely reflect the degree of nerve damage that has occurred

---

Patient-reported outcomes are becoming increasingly important to provide a comprehensive assessment of chemotherapy-induced neuropathy significance and severity. Perhaps not surprisingly, patients report significantly greater neuropathy than is reported by clinicians.

Patient-reported outcomes provide an accurate assessment of neuropathy. Accordingly, several patient questionnaires are now available, including the European Organization for Research and Treatment of Cancer (EORTC) QLQ-CIPN20 questionnaire, the Functional Assessment of Cancer/Gynecologic Oncology Group- Neurotoxicity (FACT/GOG-Ntx) questionnaire, and the Patient Neurotoxicity Questionnaire (PNQ). In addition, future versions of the National Cancer Institute (NCI) scale will include patient assessment components.

The FACT/GOG-Ntx is a questionnaire comprising 12 neuropathy-related questions and has been validated with excellent internal consistency. The questionnaire strongly correlates with measures of daily functioning, quality of life and objective neuropathy. The questionnaire also provides greater sensitivity, with each increase in NCI grade corresponding to a 4- to 6-point worsening on the FACT/GOG-Ntx scale.

Source: Park, SB et al (2013) Chemotherapy-Induced Peripheral Neurotoxicity: A Critical Analysis. CA: A Cancer Journal for Clinicians, 63:419-37. doi: 10.1002/caac.21204

4. The recommendations below

    A   Must be adjusted to each patient's individual circumstances

    B   Must be adhered to by clinicians treating anyone with osteoporosis

    C   Must be followed in order to effectively treat osteoporosis

---

Recommendations to Clinicians Treating Patients with Osteoporosis:

- Counsel on the risk of osteoporosis and related fractures.
- Advise on a diet that includes adequate amounts of total calcium intake (1000 mg/day for men 50–70; 1200 mg/day for women 51 and older and men 71 and older), incorporating dietary supplements if diet is insufficient.
- Advise on vitamin D intake (800–1000 IU/day), including supplements if necessary for individuals age 50 and older.
- Recommend regular weight-bearing and muscle- strengthening exercise to improve agility, strength, posture, and balance; maintain or improve bone strength; and reduce the risk of falls and fractures.
- Assess risk factors for falls and offer appropriate modifications (e.g. home safety assessment, balance training exercises, correction of vitamin D insufficiency, avoidance of central nervous system depressant medications, careful monitoring of antihypertensive medication, and visual correction when needed).
- Advise on cessation of tobacco smoking and avoidance of excessive alcohol intake.

Source: Cosman, F et al (2014) Clinician's Guide to Prevention and Treatment of Osteoporosis. *Osteoporosis International*, 25:2359-81. doi: 10.1007/s00198-014-2794-2

5. Health workers might help prevent antimicrobial resistance by

    A   Implementing stewardship programmes specific to their workplace

    B   Implementing stewardship programmes in primary health settings

    C   Implementing stewardship programmes covering humans and animals

Antimicrobial stewardship (AMS) refers to coordinated actions designed to promote and increase the appropriate use of antimicrobials and is a key strategy to conserve the effectiveness of antibiotics. In health care settings, AMS programmes have been shown to improve the appropriateness of antibiotic use; reduce institutional rates of resistance, morbidity and mortality; reduce health care costs, including pharmacy costs; and reduce the adverse consequences of antibiotic use, including toxicity. AMS programmes do not currently exist for all settings in which antibiotics are used. Setting-specific, evidence-based guidelines and other resources and approaches are needed to encourage the development and implementation of AMS in primary health care settings, residential aged care facilities, kennels and catteries, veterinary practices, aquaculture and farms.

Stewardship programmes covering antibiotic use in animals and food production may have significant public health value in preventing the emergence of resistant strains and their spread to humans.

Source: Australian Government (2015) National Antimicrobial Resistance Strategy 2015-2019. Published June 2015. Online ISBN: 978-1-76007-192-9.

6. The main message of the text is that

    A   Physical activity is risky and should be undertaken with caution

    B   Children should be discouraged from sports that can cause injury

    C   People should not avoid physical activity due to perceived risks

Health risks of physical activity

Concerns about safety may be a barrier to participation in some sports, particularly among children. A survey of parents in NSW identified that more than one quarter of parents of active children aged 5-12 years reported discouraging or preventing children from playing a particular sport because of injury and safety concerns. While some sports are offered to children in a modified format, which increases safety, other sport and leisure time activities could also be modified to increase participant safety.

For adults, there are some forms of physical activity that have increased rates of injury. In some instances, safety equipment may be used to reduce risk of injury. There are also risks associated with participation in too much exercise, particularly among those who have previously been sedentary. However, the benefits largely outweigh the risks, and efforts should be made to encourage participation.

Source: Australian Medical Association (2014) Physical activity position statement. Accessed from: https://ama.com.au/position-statement/physical-activity-2014

Part C

In this part of the test, there are two texts about different aspects of healthcare. For **questions 7 to 22**, choose the answer (**A**, **B**, **C** or **D**) which you think fits best according to the text.

Text 1: Asbestosis

'Asbestos' refers to a group of naturally-occurring mineral fibres composed of hydrated magnesium silicates. It was popular in commercial construction and was widely integrated into NSW homes between 1960-70. Asbestos inhalation can cause asbestosis, lung cancer and mesothelioma, with an increased risk associated with higher exposure.

Those particularly at risk of asbestos inhalation include people working in asbestos mining or milling, those who make or install asbestos products and the immediate families of these workers. Exposure to asbestos may also occur in the worker's home due to dust that has accumulated on the worker's clothing. Additionally, large quantities of asbestos still remain in buildings that were built prior to the restriction of asbestos use that applies in many countries. The weathering and aging of such buildings may cause asbestos fragments to be released in the air and create a potential hazard to building occupants.

When asbestos is released into the air, inhaled asbestos fibres enter the lungs. The foreign bodies (asbestos fibers) cause the activation of the lungs' local immune system and provoke an inflammatory reaction. Over time, chronic inflammation leads to scar formation, also known as fibrosis. The scarring of lung tissue resulting from the inhalation of asbestos fibers is specifically known as asbestosis. The scarring causes alveolar walls to thicken, which reduces elasticity and gas diffusion, reducing oxygen transfer to the blood as well as the removal of carbon dioxide. This can result in shortness of breath, a common symptom exhibited by individuals with asbestosis.

There is no cure available for asbestosis, but symptoms can be relieved with treatment. Oxygen therapy at home is often necessary to reduce shortness of breath and correct underlying low blood oxygen levels. Supportive management includes respiratory physiotherapy to remove secretions from the lungs by postural drainage, chest percussion, and vibration. Nebulized medications may be prescribed in order to loosen secretions or treat underlying chronic obstructive pulmonary disease.

In addition to asbestosis, exposure to asbestos is associated with all major histological types of lung cancer (adenocarcinoma, squamous cell carcinoma, large-cell carcinoma and small-cell carcinoma). The latency period between exposure and development of lung cancer is 20 to 30 years. It is estimated that 3%-8% of all lung cancers are related to asbestos. The risk of developing lung cancer depends on the level, duration, and frequency of asbestos exposure (cumulative exposure).

The industrial use of asbestos was banned in Australia by 2003, but not before its widespread use left a legacy of in-situ asbestos in our built environment. Currently, about one third of Australian homes contain asbestos, mostly in the form of bonded asbestos cement materials. Generally speaking, houses built before 1987 are likely to contain asbestos, especially in the eaves, internal and external wall cladding, ceilings (particularly in wet areas such as bathrooms and laundries) and fences. Caution must be exercised if these houses are to be renovated.

When asbestos is suspected of being present in building materials, it is important to have the materials tested by a qualified laboratory. Visual inspection alone is not enough to identify the presence of asbestos. However, such testing may not be warranted if the material is in good condition, in which case it is best to leave it in place. If you are carrying out maintenance such as painting or sealing on suspected asbestos-containing surfaces without sanding, wire brushing or scraping (i.e. you are not releasing any asbestos fibres into the air), you only need to take the usual precautions for these activities (such as working in a ventilated area). If the material is damaged, or will be disturbed during normal household activities or remodeling, it should be professionally tested.

Worldwide, Australia has the highest reported incidence per-capita of asbestos-related disease. Asbestos-related disease has killed thousands of Australians. An increasing number of new cases are being found in people who were exposed to asbestos fibres whilst renovating homes that were built during the period when asbestos-containing products were widely used. It is estimated that up to 25,000 more Australians will die from asbestos-related mesothelioma over the next 40 years. Thus, the effects of exposure to asbestos will need to be managed for many years to come.

Text 1: Questions 7 to 14

7. According to the first paragraph,
    A Asbestos has been used in Australia since the 1950s.
    B Inhaling naturally occurring fibre can lead to asbestosis.
    C Asbestos causes harm by increasing our exposure to mesothelioma.
    D Many of the commercially-constructed buildings built in 1960 contain asbestos.

8. People are most likely to be exposed to asbestos inhalation when…
    A Working in the coal mining industry.
    B Renovating buildings constructed prior to the restriction of its use.
    C Living with people who install asbestos products.
    D They have comorbidities that increase their risk of asbestosis exposure.

9. Regarding the mechanism of damage caused by asbestos fibres…
    A The fibres cause a prolonged inflammatory reaction in alveoli.
    B Some forms can penetrate more deeply into the lungs than others.
    C Fibres that reach the alveoli cause oxygen transfer into the blood.
    D The immune system is unable to respond to inhaled fibres.

10. Which of the following would be the best heading for the fourth paragraph?
    A Palliative treatment options for patients with asbestosis.
    B Improving the quality of life for patients with asbestosis.
    C Supportive management of shortness of breath due to asbestosis.
    D Treatment of chronic obstructive pulmonary disease.

11. According to the fifth paragraph,
    A Asbestos inhalation can cause skin tumours such as squamous cell carcinoma.
    B Exposure to asbestos fibres can cause lung cancer 30 years later.
    C Cigarette smoking causes a larger proportion of lung cancers than asbestosis.
    D Frequency of exposure to asbestos can predict the risk of lung cancer developing.

12. The presence of asbestos in Australian homes…
    A Was eliminated after a ban on the industrial use of asbestos from 2003.
    B Is only a concern in houses that are to be renovated.
    C Left a legacy of using asbestos in the construction industry.
    D Is most likely if the home was constructed prior to 1987.

13. Regarding testing for the presence of asbestos, which of the following is most correct?

    A Materials that are suspected to contain asbestos should always be tested.

    B Visual inspection can be used to determine if further testing is necessary.

    C The best course of action is to leave the suspected material in place.

    D Household activities may determine the necessity of testing.

14. What is the main reason why asbestos is a concern in Australia?

    A On average, 500 people a year will die due to asbestos exposure.

    B 25,000 Australians are currently diagnosed with asbestos-related mesothelioma.

    C There is an increasing incidence of asbestos-related disease.

    D It has the highest number of people with asbestos-related disease worldwide.

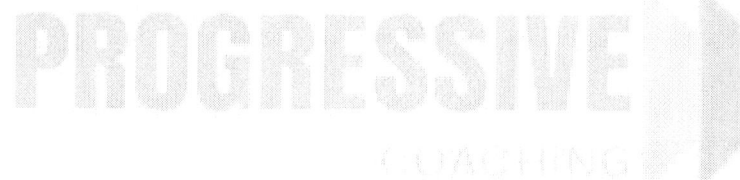

Text 2: Treatments for Epilepsy

Epileptic seizures are estimated to affect approximately 5 in every 1000 children. They have a significant impact on childhood development, with 15 to 25% of cases associated with some form of developmental delay. Early intervention to resolve seizures lasting greater than 5 minutes is recommended under a recent set of US guidelines based on a systematic review of available literature. However, anti-epileptic drugs (AEDs) have a significant adverse effect profile, and therefore it is imperative to weigh the benefits of treatment with its risks.

Benzodiazepines are the most effective and most highly studied form of acute seizure treatment with relatively few severe adverse effects aside from respiratory depression and temporary cognitive impairment. Whilst appropriate in an acute setting, long term development of tolerance (reducing its effect over time) and eventually dependence with serial use means that frequent or prolonged use is not appropriate.

Midazolam is an appropriate choice in many cases. It is a proven, efficacious treatment. A single dose resolves 70% of seizures lasting more than 5 minutes by 10 minutes, which is equivalent to the effects of diazepam and lorazepam, and more efficacious than other agents including sodium valproate or phenytoin. Especially in the context of a prehospital setting, intranasal midazolam produces results equivalent to other routes of administration that does not necessitate obtaining time-consuming IV access. In addition, it has a short half-life of 2 to 7 hours which is less than half of other comparable benzodiazepines due to its water solubility at physiological pH, reducing the duration of adverse effects.

Neuronal action potentials depend on a rapid influx of sodium through voltage-gated sodium channels to cause depolarization. Carbamazepine stabilises these channels in their inactive state, thereby reducing the ability of sodium to influx into a neuron – hence it reduces their excitability and reduces the risk of the uncontrolled electrical activity that characterises a seizure. Sodium valproate and phenytoin also have a similar function of voltage-gated sodium channel blockade – the full mechanism of sodium valproate is not fully understood, and is hypothesized to additionally increase levels of GABA within the central nervous system.

Few high-quality studies exist on the efficacy of carbamazepine on childhood epilepsy compared to placebo. Of those that do exist, many have small sample sizes leading to lower power. One study suggests that approximately 45% of children become seizure free after commencing carbamazepine. The majority of studies regarding carbamazepine are comparative studies with other AEDs. These show similar efficacy compared to sodium valproate, phenytoin and topiramate. There is still no unequivocally 'best' first-choice AED for generalised seizures in children.

AEDs including carbamazepine come with a significant profile of adverse effects, especially cognitive, due to their mechanism of action that reduces neuronal activity. One survey revealed that carbamazepine therapy produced sedative effects in 43% of the study population, ataxia in 20%, other CNS disturbances such as vertigo in 17% and negative behavioural changes in 5%. Other effects include nausea and skin rash. Only 30% reported no side effects. Measures can be taken to reduce these effects – the primary being to split the dose to twice a day to reduce the peak concentration of the medication. Carbamazepine also has significant drug interactions which must be taken into account, including accelerating the hepatic metabolism of other lipid soluble drugs, including the OCP and sodium valproate.

Patients and their families often receive education about epilepsy via outreach, including basic seizure first aid. This simple, non-pharmacological approach slightly improved quality of life outcomes in a US study. More importantly perhaps, those with greater health literacy were also found to be more compliant with medications, which may lead to better long-term outcomes. Unfortunately, little evidence exists as to long-term prognostic outcomes of epilepsy education.

Text 2: Questions 15 to 22

15. Seizures caused by epilepsy…
     A   Should be treated only if they last more than 5 minutes.
     B   Occur in around 0.5% of children.
     C   Cause developmental delay in up to 25% of children.
     D   Can be caused by developmental problems.

16. The effectiveness of benzodiazepines…
     A   Means that their dose needs to be reduced over time.
     B   Makes them inappropriate for repeated use.
     C   Is outweighed by serious side effects, such as respiratory depression.
     D   Leads to some patients taking them even when they are not having seizures.

17. Which of the following is MOST true about midazolam?
     A   It is excreted relatively quickly by the body.
     B   The adverse effects are less severe than other benzodiazepines.
     C   It can effectively stop the majority of seizures.
     D   It has similar effectiveness to sodium valproate and phenytoin.

18. Which of the following paragraphs would this be an appropriate heading for: "Treating seizures by reducing neuronal activity"?
     A   Paragraph 2
     B   Paragraph 4
     C   Paragraph 5
     D   Paragraph 7

19. What does the author suggest in the sixth paragraph regarding the AEDs that are currently available?
     A   The current evidence is insufficient to make any one AED preferable over the others.
     B   Carbamazepine is comparative to other AEDs.
     C   There are insufficient studies comparing carbamazepine to placebo.
     D   Carbamazepine can be expected to work in about half of children.

20. Regarding the side effects of AEDs, which of the following is NOT true?

    A One study found that 70% of people taking carbamazepine experienced side effects.

    B Carbamazepine can speed up the clearance of some other medications.

    C The side effects can be reduced by adjusting the dosing regime.

    D The most common side effects of carbamazepine are ataxia, vertigo and negative behavioural changes.

21. What is the most significant effect of educational interventions?

    A Improved quality of life for people with epilepsy.

    B Improved health literacy amongst epileptic patients.

    C Increased medication compliance in health-literate patients.

    D Better long-term outcomes for epileptic patients.

22. Which of the following would be the best alternative title for this text?

    A Treatment considerations in children with epilepsy.

    B The pharmacology of various epileptic treatments.

    C The use of benzodiazepines in epilepsy.

    D Challenges in the management of epilepsy.

Test 3: Answer Key

Part A

Questions 1 to 20

1	B
2	C
3	D
4	A
5	D
6	A
7	D
8	potassium chloride
9	via nasogastric tube
10	additional intravenous fluids
11	infants and young children
12	village health workers
13	small intestine
14	2-3 years
15	tropical countries
16	not prolonged
17	small but significant
18	glucose
19	combined with
20	highly suited

Part B

Questions 1 to 6

1	B	Put patient care above their students' educational needs
2	C	Identify the greatest level of disability for the patient being tested
3	C	Closely reflect the degree of nerve damage that has occurred
4	A	Must be adjusted to each patient's individual circumstances
5	A	Implementing stewardship programmes specific to their workplace
6	C	People should not avoid physical activity due to perceived risks

Part C

Questions 7 to 14

7	D	Many of the commercially-constructed buildings built in 1960 contain asbestos.
8	C	Living with people who install asbestos products.
9	A	The fibres cause a prolonged inflammatory reaction in alveoli.
10	A	Palliative treatment options for patients with asbestosis.
11	B	Exposure to asbestos fibres can cause lung cancer 30 years later.
12	D	Is most likely if the home was constructed prior to 1987.
13	D	Household activities may determine the necessity of testing.
14	A	On average, 500 people a year will die due to asbestos exposure.

Questions 15 to 22

15	B	Occur in around 0.5% of children.
16	D	Leads to some patients taking them even when they are not having seizures.
17	A	It is excreted relatively quickly by the body.
18	C	Paragraph 5
19	A	The current evidence is insufficient to make any one AED preferable over the others.
20	D	The most common side effects of carbamazepine are ataxia, vertigo and negative behavioural changes.
21	C	Increased medication compliance in health-literate patients.
22	A	Treatment considerations in children with epilepsy.

END OF KEY

Test 3: Answer Guide

Part A

Diarrhoea 4 l Oral Rehydration Therapy
Acute diarr.....al diseases are one of the leading causes of mortality in infants and young children 11 any developing countries. In most cases, death is caused by dehydration.
Dehydration from diarrhoea can be prevented 6 jiving extra fluids at home, or it can be treated simply, effectively, and cheaply in all age-groups and in all but the most severe cases by giving patients by mouth an adequate glucose-electrolyte solution.
This way of giving fluids to prevent or treat dehydration is called oral rehydration therapy (ORT). ORT, combined with 19 ance on appropriate feeding practices, is the main strategy recommended by t.... WHO Department of Child and Adolescent Health and Development (CAH) to achieve a reduction in diarrhoea-related mortality and malnutrition in children.
Oral rehydration therapy (ORT) can be delivered by village health workers 12 practiced in t'.... ome by mothers with some guidance, and thus is a technology highly suited 20 ie primary health care approach.

TABL 1 Composition of the new ORS formulation

New ORS	grams/litre	%	New ORS	mmol/litre
Sodium chloride	2.6	12.683	Sodium	75
Glucose, anhydrous	13.5	65.854 18	Chloride	65
Potassium chloride	1.5 8	7.317	Glucose, anhydrous	75
Trisodium citrate, dihydrate	2.9	14.146	Potassium	20
			Citrate	10
Total	**20.5**	**100.00**	**Total Osmolarity**	**245**

Text C

Abstract: Replacement of Water and Electrolyte Losses 2 Cholera by an Oral Glucose-Electrolyte Solution (Pierce et al, 1969)

Background: The efficacy of an orally administered glucose-electrolyte solution in replacing stool losses of water and electrolytes in severe cholera was evaluated.

Methods: After initial intravenous rehydration, intravenous fluids were discontinued, and subsequent water and electrolyte losses were replaced by the oral solution administered via nasogastric tube 9

Results: In 9 of 10 patients so treated, water, electrolyte, and acid-base balances were adequately maintained by this method until diarrhoea ended. One patient with very severe diarrhoea required small amounts of additional intravenous fluids 10 maintain water balance. Patients receiving the oral solution h 17 small but significant increase in stool output during oral fluid administra..... when compared with the 10 patients in the control group who received only intravenous replacement of stool losses. Calculated absorption of the oral fluid was 87%.

Conclusion: Duration of diarrhoea and of VIBRIO CHOLERAE excretion 16 not prolonged by the oral solution administration. The role of glucose in the absorption of water and sodium by the small bowel is discussed. The study suggests a useful role for such an orally administered glucose-electrolyte solution in the management of cholera.

Text D

Therapeutic Mechanisms 3 ORS

The pharmacokinetics and ....chanisms of therapeutic action of the substances in the ORS solution are as follows:

- Glucose facilitates the abs.......on of sodium (and hence water) on a 1:1 molar 13 basis in the small intestine
- Sodium and potassium are needed 7 replace the body losses of these essential ions during diarrhoea (and vomiting).
- 5 Citrate corrects the acidosis that occurs as a result of diarrhoea and dehydration. The particular advantage of citrate containing ORS (over bicarbonate containing ORS) is its stabili 15 tropical countries where temperatures up to 60°C can occur. A shelf-life of 2-3 years 14 be assumed without any particular storage precautions.

Part B

1. Healthcare workers who are in a teaching position should
   - A Incorrect: The adjective "own" emphasises that the patient is responsible for maintaining their comfort and dignity, but the text does not suggest exactly who is responsible.
   - **B Correct: This is emphasised in the second and third points, where patient treatment and comfort are prioritised first.**
   - C Incorrect: This is not referred to in the text.

2. The grading system below aims to
   - A Incorrect: Daily functions, such as dressing and showering oneself, are not necessarily reflected in individual movements and can be affected by adaptive and assistive devices.
   - B Incorrect: The grading system focuses on the least level of functioning, as per the explanation for answer C.
   - **C Correct: The score is defined by "the weakest muscle in each group", which is the most disabled.**

3. Patient-reported outcomes
   - A Incorrect: The response of clinicians to patient-reported outcomes is not stated.
   - B Incorrect: The text does not refer to the frequency of cases where outcomes are different to the degree of neuropathy (stage of their condition).
   - **C Correct: This is stated throughout the text: "an accurate assessment of neuropathy" and "strongly correlates with...objective neuropathy."**

4. The recommendations below
   - **A Correct: Differences in the recommendations are presented based on the patient's gender, age and risk factors.**
   - B Incorrect: This answer is too strong, as they are recommendations, not requirements.
   - C Incorrect: This answer implies that osteoporosis cannot be effectively treated in any other way, which is beyond the scope of the information in the text.

5. Health workers might help prevent antimicrobial resistance by
   - **A Correct: The text states that "Setting-specific, evidence-based guidelines and other resources and approaches are needed..."**
   - B Incorrect: This is not the case for health workers who are not located in primary health settings.
   - C Incorrect: This is not relevant for health workers who either don't work with humans or don't work with animals.

6. The main message of the text is that
   - A Incorrect: While this is not contradicted by the text, it is not the entire main message being conveyed.
   - B Incorrect: The text simply reports that one quarter of parents do this.
   - **C Correct: The text describes concerns in the community about the risks of physical activity and how these might be addressed and concludes by stating that "the benefits outweigh the risks".**

Part C

7. According to the first paragraph,
    - **A** Incorrect: the text only says that it was "widely integrated into NSW homes between 1960-70". It may have been used *prior to* the 1950s.
    - **B** Incorrect: the term "naturally occurring fibre" is too broad, as it could also refer to the fibre in plants. The text only refers to asbestos, not *all* naturally-occurring fibre.
    - **C** Incorrect: The text states that asbestos can cause mesothelioma.
    - **D** **Correct: This is referred to in the text: "was widely integrated into NSW homes between 1960-70". Homes are included in commercially-constructed buildings, as they are built to be sold for profit.**

8. People are most likely to be exposed to asbestos inhalation when…
    - **A** Incorrect: the text refers to "asbestos mining", not coal mining.
    - **B** Incorrect: This is too general. Renovating buildings whilst following the correct precautions and protocols is unlikely to lead to asbestos exposure.
    - **C** **Correct: this is referred to in the text as "the immediate families of these workers".**
    - **D** Incorrect: Comorbidities that increase people's risk of exposure to asbestos are not referred to in the text.

9. Regarding the mechanism of damage caused by asbestos fibres…
    - **A** **Correct: this is referred to in the text: "foreign bodies (asbestos fibers) cause the activation of the lungs' local immune system… this reaction becomes chronic".**
    - **B** Incorrect: the text doesn't state that different fibres penetrate more deeply than others, but simply that "All forms of asbestos fibers are able to penetrate deeply into the lower respiratory tract".
    - **C** Incorrect: The text only states that alveoli are "where oxygen is transferred into the blood".
    - **D** Incorrect: The immune system *does* respond ("cause the activation of the lungs' local immune system and provoke an inflammatory reaction"), just not effectively.

10. Which of the following would be the best heading for the fifth paragraph?
    - **A** **Correct: This option reflects the topic sentence of the paragraph (relief of symptoms) as well as the body (methods of symptom relief). Since palliative treatment is treatment which focusses on symptom relief and providing comfort care, this is the best heading.**
    - **B** Incorrect: This is not directly discussed in the paragraph. Symptom relief may improve quality of life secondarily, but quality of life also includes other factors such as living arrangements, nutrition and social functioning, which aren't discussed.
    - **C** Incorrect: This is only one of the details mentioned in the paragraph, so it would not make a good heading. A heading should summarise the main idea/topic presented in a paragraph.

D Incorrect: This is only one of the details mentioned in the paragraph, so it would not make a good heading. A heading should summarise the main idea/topic presented in a paragraph.

11. According to the sixth paragraph,

A Incorrect: Squamous cell carcinoma is listed as a type of lung cancer, not skin tumour.

B Correct: This is stated in the text: "The latency period between exposure and development of lung cancer is 20 to 30 years".

C Incorrect: The proportion of lung cancer caused by cigarette smoking is not mentioned in the text, and you are being asked to choose the correct option *according to paragraph 6*, so this is not the correct choice.

D Incorrect: Frequency is only one factor involved ("The risk of developing lung cancer depends on the level, duration, and frequency") so it cannot predict the risk of lung cancer unless the level and duration of exposure are also known.

12. The presence of asbestos in Australian homes...

A Incorrect: The ban stopped further industrial use of asbestos, but this doesn't mean that asbestos already present in homes was removed.

B Incorrect: This option is too narrow. The text does state that "Caution must be exercised if these houses are to be renovated." However, this doesn't mean that asbestos is not a concern in other situations.

C Incorrect: The verb "using" makes this option wrong. The text only states that the use of asbestos "left a legacy of in-situ asbestos", that is, it left behind asbestos that had already been put in place.

D Correct: This answer is closest to what is stated in the text: "houses built before 1987 are likely to contain asbestos".

13. Regarding testing for the presence of asbestos, which of the following is most correct?

A Incorrect: The text states that "such testing may not be warranted if the material is in good condition".

B Incorrect: In regard to visual inspection, the text only states that "Visual inspection alone is not enough to identify the presence of asbestos."

C Incorrect: According to the text, this is only true "if the material is in good condition".

D Correct: This is referred to in the text: "If the material...will be disturbed during normal household activities or remodeling, it should be professionally tested."

14. What is the main reason why asbestos is a concern in Australia?

A Correct: The text states that "It is estimated that up to 25,000 more Australians will die from asbestos-related mesothelioma over the next 40 years." This is an average of 500 people per year over the next 40 years.

B Incorrect: The text only states that "25,000 more Australians will die", not that they are diagnosed.

C Incorrect: The text only states that "An increasing number of new cases are being found in people who were exposed to asbestos fibres whilst renovating homes". The overall incidence is not stated.

D Incorrect: The text states that "Australia has the highest reported *incidence* per-capita of asbestos-related disease". This is not the same as "the highest number".

15. Seizures caused by epilepsy...

A Incorrect: The text does state that "Early intervention to resolve seizures lasting greater than 5 minutes is recommended", but this doesn't mean that no treatment should be given for seizures lasting less than 5 minutes.

B Correct: The text states "approximately 5 in every 1000 children" which is the same as 0.5%.

C Incorrect: The text states that "15-25% of cases associated with some form of developmental delay", but not that seizures are the cause of this delay.

D Incorrect: The text states that "15-25% of cases associated with some form of developmental delay", but not that seizures can lead to this delay.

16. The effectiveness of benzodiazepines...

A Incorrect: The text states that "frequent or prolonged use is not appropriate" but not that the dose needs to be reduced over time.

B Incorrect: The text states that "frequent or prolonged use is not appropriate" but not that they cannot be used repeatedly for *short* periods of time.

C Incorrect: This means that the adverse effects are more important than the effectiveness, which is not stated in the text. In fact, the text states that benzodiazepines are "appropriate in an acute setting", which contradicts this answer option.

D Correct: The text states that benzodiazepines have a "long term development of tolerance...and eventually dependence". Since dependence means addiction to a drug, this answer is correct.

17. Which of the following is MOST true about midazolam?

A Correct: This is stated in the text ("it has a short half-life of 2-7 hours which is less than half of other comparable benzodiazepines"). The "half-life" means the time in which half of the drug can be removed from the blood by the body.

B Incorrect: The text states that the short half-life of midazolam reduces "the *duration* of adverse effects", not the *severity*.

C Incorrect: The text only states that "a single dose resolves 70% of seizures *lasting more than 5 minutes*". These seizures may still constitute a minority of seizures overall.

D Incorrect: The text states that midazolam is "*more* efficacious than other agents including sodium valproate or phenytoin", so this answer is inaccurate.

18. Which of the following paragraphs would this be an appropriate heading for: "Treating seizures by reducing neuronal activity"?

    A Incorrect: This paragraph only covers the mechanism of action of benzodiazepines, one class of drugs used to treat seizures. Therefore, it is too specific for the proposed heading.

    B Incorrect: This paragraph describes midazolam and doesn't mention neuronal activity. Therefore, it is not suitable for the proposed heading.

    C **Correct: The heading summarises this paragraph well and refers to the content of the topic sentence ("Neuronal action potentials") and concluding sentence ("function of voltage-gated sodium channel blockade") in the paragraph. Therefore, this is the best choice.**

    D Incorrect: This paragraph focuses mainly on the adverse effects of AEDs. Therefore, the proposed heading would not be an appropriate summary.

19. What does the author suggest in the sixth paragraph regarding the AEDs that are currently available?

    A **Correct: This is referred to in the text by the phrases "Few high-quality studies exist", "Of those that do exist, many have small sample sizes leading to lower power" and "there is still no unequivocally 'best' first-choice AED".**

    B Incorrect: The text does state that studies have shown carbamazepine has "*similar efficacy* compared to sodium valproate, phenytoin and topiramate", but this doesn't mean the same as "comparative". In fact, the word "comparative" is being used to describe the studies.

    C Incorrect: The author is stating that there are insufficient *high-quality* studies comparing carbamazepine to placebo. This is slightly different to saying that there are too few studies in general.

    D Incorrect: This is one of the results that the author reports ("One study suggests that approximately 45% of children become seizure free") but this is a fact, not a suggestion.

20. Regarding the side effects of AEDs, which of the following is NOT true?

    A Incorrect: The text does state this ("Only 30% reported no side effects"). Since this is true according to the text, it is not the correct choice.

    B Incorrect: The text does state this ("accelerating the hepatic metabolism of other lipid soluble drugs"). Since this is true according to the text, it is not the correct choice.

    C Incorrect: The text does state this ("Measures can be taken to reduce these effects – the primary being to split the dose to twice a day"). Since this is true according to the text, it is not the correct choice.

    D **Correct: The text actually states that sedative effects, ataxia and vertigo are the most common side effects ("sedative effects in 43% of the study population, ataxia in 20%, other CNS disturbances such as vertigo in 17%"). Since this answer contradicts the text, it is the correct choice.**

21. What is the most significant effect of educational interventions?

    A Incorrect: The text states that these interventions only had a minor effect on quality of life ("slightly improved quality of life outcomes").

B Incorrect: The text actually refers to health literacy in order to describe the group that improved their compliance ("those with greater health literacy were also found to be more compliant with medications"). This doesn't mean the same as improving health literacy.

C **Correct: This is supported by the sentence:** *"More importantly perhaps, those with greater health literacy were also found to be more compliant* **with medications, which may lead to** *better long-term outcomes."*

D Incorrect: This is unclear according to the text, since the author states that "little evidence exists as to long-term prognostic outcomes of epilepsy education."

22. Which of the following would be the best alternative title for this text?

A **Correct: This title provides a good summary of the text. It is referred to in parts of the introduction ("Epileptic seizures are estimated to affect approximately 5 in every 1000 children...it is imperative to weigh the benefits of treatment with its risks"), body ("suitable for use in an acute seizure setting", "long term development of tolerance", "more efficacious than other agents", etc.) and conclusion ("non-pharmacological approach slightly improved quality of life" and "better long-term outcomes").**

B Incorrect: This option only refers to a part of the text and doesn't include other issues described, such as effectiveness, adverse effects and patient education.

C Incorrect: This option is very specific, as it focuses on benzodiazepines. It doesn't refer to other anti-epileptic drugs and treatments which are discussed in the text.

D Incorrect: This option is also quite specific, as it doesn't cover other topics discussed in the text, such as the pharmacology, adverse effects and effectiveness of anti-epileptic drugs.

Notes

Notes

30737329R00067

Printed in Poland
by Amazon Fulfillment
Poland Sp. z o.o., Wrocław